Essential Nurse Prescribing

Essential Nurse Prescribing

Molly Courtenay
PhD MSc BSc RGN RNT CertEd
Lecturer, School of Nursing and Midwifery
University of Southampton

Michele Butler
MmedSci BSc (Hons) RGN RNT CertEd (FE)
Senior Lecturer in Clinical Science
Oxford Brookes University

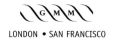

LONDON • SAN FRANCISCO

GMM

www.greenwich-medical.co.uk

© 2002
Greenwich Medical Media Limited
137 Euston Road
London
NW1 2AA

870 Market Street, Ste 720
San Francisco
CA 94102

ISBN 1 84110 108 7

First Published 2002

Design by Bright Yellow Design & Marketing

Typeset by Mizpah Publishing Services, Chennai, India

Printed in the UK by the Alden Group, Oxford

Distributed by Plymbridge Distributors Ltd and in the USA by Jamco Distribution

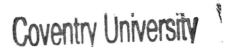

CONTENTS

PREFACE

Nurses working in the expanded role of prescriber will frequently be faced with prescribing decisions. This text provides easily accessible information upon which to base these decisions, ensuring safe and effective prescribing practices. Each chapter examines preparations available to nurses in the extended formulary and their effects on the human body. These preparations can be prescribed in the following four areas:

- Minor ailments
- Minor injuries
- Health promotion
- Palliative care

Information including product dosage, contraindications, adverse effects, drug interactions, and specific nursing points is presented in detail. This text adopts the same approach as Nurse Prescribing: Principles and Practice, written by the same authors, in that it provides key background information from the relevant life sciences, as it applies to modern clinical practice.

The authors have brought together widely available information in the form of a single, easy to use, practice based text, which, in conjunction with the NPF/BNF, Drug Tariff and manufacturers' product information sheets, provides an essential guide to nurse prescribing.

M.C.
M.B.
May 2002

Introduction

In 1986, recommendations were made for nurses to take on the role of prescribing. The Cumberlege Report *Neighbourhood Nursing: A Focus for Care* (Department of Health and Social Security (DHSS), 1986), examined the care given to patients in their homes by district nurses (DNs) and health visitors (HVs). It was identified that some very complicated procedures had arisen around prescribing in the community, and that nurses were wasting their time requesting prescriptions from the general practitioner (GP) for such items as wound dressings and ointments. The report suggested that patient care could be improved, and resources used more effectively, if community nurses were able to prescribe, as part of their everyday nursing practice, from a limited list of items and simple agents agreed by the DHSS.

During 1989 a report was published which made a number of recommendations involving the categories of items for which nurses might prescribe, together with the circumstances under which they might be prescribed (Department of Health (DoH), 1989). The report suggested that a number of benefits would occur as a result of nurses adopting the role of prescriber. As well as improved patient care, this included improved use of both patients' and nurses' time and improved communication between team members.

During 1992, the primary legislation permitting nurses to prescribe a limited range of drugs was passed (Medicinal Products: Prescribing by Nurses Act 1992). The necessary amendments were made to this act in 1994 and a revised list of products available to the nurse prescriber was published in the Nurse Prescribers' Formulary (NPF) (see Table I.1).

Following the success of demonstration sites, pilot sites were set up in England for nurse prescribing. Evaluation of these pilot schemes was positive, and the funding for full national implementation of nurse prescribing was promised by former Health Secretary Frank Dobson at the Royal College of Nursing conference in April 1998. By the spring of 2001, over 20,000 DNs and HVs (including some practice nurses) were qualified prescribers. Additionally, post registration programmes for DNs and HVs included the necessary educational component qualifying nurses to prescribe.

In 1999, it was recommended that prescribing authority should be extended to other groups of professionals with training and expertise in specialised areas (DoH, 1999). During 2001 support was given by the Government for this extension (DoH, 2001), and funding was made available for other nurses, as well as those currently qualified to prescribe, to undergo the necessary training to enable them to prescribe from an extended formulary. This formulary includes:

- All General Sales List (GSL) items, i.e. those that can be sold to the public without the supervision of a pharmacist.

Table I.1 – Items in the NPF

- Laxatives
- Analgesics
- Local anaesthetics
- Drugs for the mouth
- Removal of ear wax
- Drugs for threadworm
- Drugs for scabies and head lice
- Skin preparations
- Disinfection and cleansing
- Wound management products
- Elastic hosiery
- Urinary catheters and appliances
- Stoma care products
- Appliances and reagents for diabetes
- Fertility and gynaecological products

(ENB, 1998).

- All Pharmacy (P) medicines, i.e. those products sold under the supervision of a pharmacist.
- A number of specified Prescription-only-Medicines (POMs), enabling nurses to prescribe in four areas, i.e. minor ailments, minor injuries, health promotion, and palliative care.

Education and training for extended nurse prescribing commenced during January 2002. Programmes are at academic level 3, involve 25 taught days, additional self-directed learning, and 12 days learning in practice with a practice supporter (a doctor), over a 3 month period.

Compared to the 'older' training, which involved an open learning pack and a 3 day taught component, this is a substantial increase in both the theoretical and practice components. However, it is important to remember the size of the 'new' formulary. Although POMs may be limited, the number (over 130) far exceeds those listed on the 'old' formulary (12 – see Table I.2). In addition to this, prescribers have access to all GSL and P preparations. Therefore, it is important that education programmes are sufficiently robust to ensure safe and effective prescribing.

It has been highlighted by studies evaluating nurse prescribing that areas in which nurses require further knowledge is pharmacology, and choice of preparation to be prescribed (Blenkinsopp *et al.*, 1998). The extension of nurse prescribing has meant that there is an increased need for this knowledge. The nurse prescriber is accountable both legally and professionally. Therefore, it is vital that they have a clear understanding of each of the products listed in the extended formulary and are able to provide a rationale for

- What is prescribed.
- When over-the-counter products are recommended.

Table I.2 – List of POMs, prescribable by DNs and HVs

Co-danthramer Capsules
Co-danthramer Capsules Strong
Co-danthramer Oral Suspension
Co-danthramer Oral Suspension Strong
Co-danthrusate Capsules
Co-danthrusate Oral Suspension
Mebendazole Tablets
Mebendazole Oral Suspension
Miconazole Oral Gel
Nystatin Oral Suspension
Nystatin Pastilles
Streptokinase and Streptodornase Topical Powder

Medicines Control Agency (MCA) 2001.

- When a decision is made not to prescribe or recommend a product (English National Board (ENB), 1998).

This knowledge must also be assessed in the context of

- The patient's circumstances including current medication.
- The patient's past medical history.
- The patient's current and anticipated health status.
- A thorough knowledge of the item to be prescribed – its therapeutic action, adverse effects, dosage, and interaction.
- A thorough knowledge of the alternatives to prescribing.
- Frequency of use in a variety of circumstances (ENB, 1998).

Furthermore, a very relevant issue for the nurse prescriber, introduced by the 'Code of Professional Conduct' (United Kingdom Central Council for Nursing, Midwifery, and Health Visiting (UKCCa) 1992) and the allied 'Scope of Professional Practice' (UKCCb, 1992), is the notion of nurse decision-making and delegation. That is, nurses are not only responsible for the care they provide but also for the care given by others, as a result of a nursing decision. Someone other than the nurse, e.g. a patient, a carer or a health care assistant, will often administer items prescribed by the nurse prescriber. However, the nurse initially writing the prescription is legally responsible for ensuring that the product is used as outlined by the instructions. For example, the nurse may delegate the responsibility of applying insecticide shampoo to a mother, or delegate the application of a barrier cream to a carer.

For the above reasons, it is essential that nurses have a thorough knowledge and understanding of pharmacology in relation to each of the products in the NPEF. This includes pharmacokinetics and pharmacodynamics.

Pharmacokinetics involves the changes in serum concentration of a drug in the body over time. Absorption, distribution, metabolism, and excretion of the drug bring this about. The last two processes also account for elimination of the drug from the body. Pharmacodynamics is the term used to describe what a drug does to the body, including both therapeutic and adverse effects. For nurses to develop their knowledge of these subjects, it is essential that they also have a sound understanding of related anatomy, physiology, and disease processes. This knowledge will enable the nurse to inform the patient of such issues as

- What to expect when prescribing a product.
- How to administer the product.
- The duration of time taken in which to see an improvement.
- The effectiveness of the product.
- Any precautions the patient should take.
- The possible likelihood of adverse effects allowing the probable cause to be recognised, and a note made in the patient's records following their occurrence (ENB, 1998).

For example, in relation to pharmacodynamics, i.e. monitoring the actions of drugs and detecting their adverse effects and interactions, if the nurse is prescribing oral analgesics, e.g. aspirin, they need to be aware of the possible adverse effects and drug interactions of this product. Adverse effects of aspirin include gastric irritation and bleeding, tinnitus, anticoagulation, hypersensitivity, liver and kidney impairment, Reyes syndrome, and foetal defects in pregnant women. Aspirin interacts with a number of drugs including anticoagulants. To fully appreciate these effects and interactions, an understanding of the action of aspirin at a cellular level is a necessary prerequisite. This knowledge will enable the nurse to identify those patient groups in which aspirin should be avoided. These would include: patients with a history of gastric problems; the elderly, as this group suffer most from this adverse effect; asthmatics as they are more likely to suffer from hypersensitivity; patients with renal and liver impairment; pregnant women, breast feeding mothers, and children under 12 years. It should also be cautioned in patients receiving a low daily dose of aspirin for the prophylaxis of cerebral vascular disease or myocardial infarction.

Similarly, an awareness of the abdominal cramping associated with stimulant laxatives would enable the nurse to warn the patient of this particularly unpleasant effect and be aware of their possible occurrence.

To fully understand the routes of administration and absorption of drugs (pharmacokinetics), anatomical, physiological, and knowledge of disease processes is also essential. For example, when prescribing topically administered medications to the elderly, it is vital that the nurse appreciates why the absorption rate of these medications decrease in this patient group. To begin to develop an understanding of this issue, they need to be aware of the physiological changes that occur to the skin as people age, such as decreased hydration, increased keratinisation, and decreased blood perfusion. To fully understand orally administered medication, knowledge of the gastrointestinal tract is crucial. Factors that effect absorption, such as pH of the absorption environment, motility of the gastrointestinal tract, the presence of food or other materials such as drugs, and the general health of the gastrointestinal mucosa, can then be fully appreciated.

It is clear, that if nurse prescribers are to prescribe safely and effectively and be accountable for their prescribing decisions, there is a need for them to develop and maintain their knowledge of pharmacology, anatomy, physiology and disease processes. This book has been developed in response to this need. It adopts a similar approach to Nurse Prescribing Principles and Practice which was written for DNs and HVs working in the role of prescriber. Readers are provided with easily accessible information which, in conjunction with the NPF/BNF, and manufacturers' product information sheets, provides an essential guide to nurse prescribing facilitating safe and effective prescribing practice. Chapters examine the pharmacology of preparations listed in the NPEF and adopt a systems approach in order to clearly link pharmacological information with anatomical and physiological knowledge. Each chapter looks at a different system of the human body, integrating information on the different conditions affecting the components of this system and the pharmacology of the products used to treat these conditions. As in *Nurse Prescribing: Principles and Practice*, the mode of action, contraindications, adverse effects, and nursing points pertaining to each preparation is outlined.

Throughout the text both generic and trade names are supplied. This format has been retained as readers of *Nurse Prescribing: Principles and Practice* found this useful.

However, the authors wish to emphasise that only the generic name should be used when writing a prescription.

References

Blenkinsopp A, Grime J, Pollock K, Boardman H (1998). *Nurse Prescribing Evaluation (1): The Initial Training programme and Implementation*. Keele University: Department of Medicines Management.

DoH (1989). *Report of the Advisory Group on Nurse Prescribing (Crown Report)*. London: DoH.

DoH (1999). *Review of Prescribing, Supply and Administration of Medicines (Crown Report)*. London: DoH.

DoH (2001). *Consultation on Proposals to Extend Nurse Prescribing*. London: DoH.

DHSS (1986). *Neighbourhood Nursing: A Focus for Care (Cumberlege Report)*. London: HMSO.

ENB (1998). *Nurse Prescribing Open Learning Pack*. Milton Keynes: Learning Materials Design.

MCA (2001). *Extended Prescribing of Prescription Only Medicines By Independent Nurse Prescribers*. London: MCA.

UKCCa (1992). *Code of Professional Conduct*. London: UKCC.

UKCCb (1992). *The Scope of Professional Practice*. London: UKCC.

Chapter 1

Basic Pharmacology

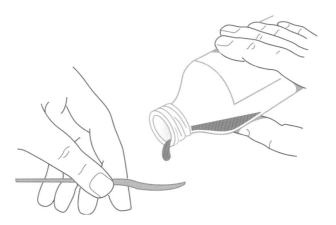

An appropriate knowledge and understanding of pharmacology is essential for the nurse prescriber. It will influence decision-making regarding the most appropriate drug, the route of administration, the dose and frequency, potential contraindications, adverse effects, and interactions with other drugs.

This chapter provides fundamental information regarding pharmacokinetics and pharmacodynamics and highlights issues that should be considered when assessing patients with respect to prescribing medication.

A list of other useful textbooks has been provided at the end of the chapter, for those nurse prescribers wishing to read further.

Routes of Administration

Drugs may act locally or systemically. Locally implies that the effects of the drug are confined to a specific area. Systemically means that the drug has to enter the vascular and lymphatic systems for delivery to body tissues. The main route of administration to provide a local effect is topical, whilst oral or parenteral administration of drugs are the main routes to provide a systemic effect. Some topical drugs can, however, have systemic effects, especially if given in large doses, in frequent doses or over a long period of time.

Topical administration

Topical preparations may be applied to the skin, mouth, nose, oropharynx, cornea, ear, urethra, vagina or rectum. These preparations may be administered in a variety of forms including:

- creams
- ointments
- gels
- lotions
- aerosols
- foams
- plasters
- powders
- patches
- suppositories
- sprays

Oral administration

This route of administration, which implies 'by mouth', is most commonly used. It tends to be convenient, simple and usually safe. Preparations may be in a solid form and include:

- tablets
- capsules
- powders
- granules
- lozenges

Other preparations may be provided in a liquid form and include:

- solutions
- emulsions
- suspensions
- syrups
- elixirs
- tinctures

Parenteral administration

Parenteral administration of a drug refers to the giving of a preparation by any route other than the gastrointestinal tract, by which a drug is injected or infused. This, therefore, includes intradermal, subcutaneous, intramuscular, intravenous, intrathecal, and intra-articular routes. These sterile preparations are presented in ampules, vials, cartridges or large-volume containers.

Pharmacokinetics

Pharmacokinetics considers the movement of drugs within the body and the way in which the body affects drugs with time. Once a drug has been administered by one of the routes previously described, it will then undergo four basic processes:

- Absorption
- Distribution
- Metabolism
- Excretion

The composition of the drug has an important influence on where the drug is absorbed, where the drug is distributed to, where and how effectively it is metabolised and finally how rapidly it is excreted. In addition, other factors such as the dose of drug, the patient's condition, and other therapeutic and environmental issues may also affect the effectiveness of these processes. Each of these processes will now be considered in more detail.

Drug absorption

The process of absorption brings the drug from the site of administration into the circulatory or lymphatic system. Almost all drugs, other than those administered intravenously or some that are applied topically, must be absorbed before they can have an effect on the body. The term *bioavailability* is used to refer to the proportion of the administered drug that has reached the circulation, and that is available to have an effect. Drugs given intravenously may be considered to be 100% bioavailable as they are administered directly into the circulation and all of the drug may potentially cause an effect.

Administration by other routes means that some of the drug molecules will be lost during absorption and distribution, and thus bioavailability is reduced.

Drugs administered orally are absorbed from the gastrointestinal tract, carried via the hepatic portal vein to the liver, and then undergo some metabolism by the liver before the drug has even had the opportunity to work. This removal of a drug by the liver, before the drug has become available for use, is called the *first pass effect*. Some drugs, when swallowed and absorbed, will be almost totally inactivated by the first pass effect, e.g. glyceryl trinitrate. The first pass effect can, however, be avoided if the drug is given by another route. Thus, glyceryl trinitrate, when administered sublingually or transdermally, avoids first pass metabolism by the liver and is able to cause a therapeutic effect.

Absorption following oral administration

For drugs given by all routes other than the intravenous route, several lipid cell membrane barriers will have to be passed before the drug reaches the circulation. Four major transport mechanisms exist to facilitate this process.

Passive diffusion is the most important and most common. If the drug is present in the gastrointestinal tract in a greater concentration that it is in the bloodstream, then a concentration gradient is said to exist. The presence of the concentration gradient will carry the drug through the cell membrane and into the circulation. The drug will be transported until the concentrations of drug are equal on either side of the cell membrane. No energy is expended during this process.

Facilitated diffusion allows low lipid-soluble drugs to be transported across the cell membrane by combining with a carrier molecule. This also requires a concentration gradient and expends no energy.

Active transport is only used by drugs which closely resemble natural body substances. This process works against a concentration gradient and requires a carrier molecule and energy to be expended.

Pinocytosis or 'cell-drinking' is not a common method for absorbing drugs. It requires energy and involves the cell membrane invaginating and engulfing a fluid-filled vesicle or sac.

Factors affecting drug absorption from the gastrointestinal tract

A number of factors may influence the absorption of a drug from the gut.

These include:

- *Gut motility* – If motility is increased and therefore transit time is reduced, there will be less time available for absorption of a drug. Hypomotility may increase the amount of drug absorbed if contact with the gut epithelium is prolonged.
- *Gastric emptying* – If increased, this will speed up drug absorption rate. If delayed, it will slow the delivery of drug to the intestine, therefore reducing the absorption rate.
- *Surface area* – The rate of drug absorption is greatest in the small intestine due to the large surface area provided by the villi.
- *Gut pH* – The pH of the gastrointestinal tract varies along its length. The changing environmental pH may have different effects on different drugs. Optimal absorption of a drug may be dependent on a specific pH.
- *Blood flow* – The small intestine has a very good blood supply which is one reason why most absorption occurs in this part of the gut. Faster absorption rates will occur in areas where blood supply is ample.
- *Presence of food and fluid in the gastrointestinal tract* – The presence of food in the gut may selectively increase or decrease drug absorption. For example, food increases the absorption of dicoumarol, whilst tetracycline absorption is reduced by the presence of dairy foods. Fluid taken with medication will aid dissolution of the drug and enhance its passage to the small intestine.
- *Antacids* – The presence of these in the gastrointestinal tract causes a change in environmental pH. They will increase absorption of basic drugs and decrease absorption of acidic ones.
- *Drug composition* – Various factors pertaining to the composition of the drug may affect the rate at which it is absorbed. For example, liquid preparations are more rapidly absorbed than solid ones, the presence of an enteric coating may slow absorption, and lipid-soluble drugs are rapidly absorbed.

Absorption following parenteral administration

Intradermal drugs diffuse slowly from the injection site into local capillaries, and the process is a little faster with drugs administered subcutaneously. Due to the rich supply of blood to muscles, absorption following an intramuscular injection is even quicker. The degree of tissue perfusion and condition of the injection site will influence the rate of drug absorption.

Absorption following topical administration

Drugs applied topically to the mucous membranes and skin are absorbed less than by oral and parenteral routes. Absorption is, however, increased if the skin is broken or if the area is covered with an occlusive dressing.

Rectal and sublingual absorption is usually rapid due to the vascularity of the mucosa. Absorption from instillation into the nose may lead to systemic as well as local effects, whilst inhalation into the lungs provides for extensive absorption. Minimal absorption will occur from instillation into the ears, but absorption from the eyes depends on whether a solution or ointment is administered.

Drug distribution

This process involves the transportation of the drug to the target site of action.

During distribution, some drug molecules may be deposited at storage sites and others may be deposited and inactivated. Various factors may influence how and even if, a drug is distributed.

- *Blood flow* – Distribution may depend on tissue perfusion. Organs that are highly vascular such as the heart, liver, and kidneys will rapidly acquire a drug. Levels of a drug in bone, fat, muscle, and skin may take some time to rise due to reduced vascularity. The patient's level of activity and local tissue temperature may also affect drug distribution to the skin and muscle.

- *Plasma protein binding* – In the circulation, a drug is bound to circulating plasma proteins or is 'free' in an un-bound state. The plasma protein usually involved in binding a drug is albumin. If a drug is bound, then it is said to be inactive and cannot have a pharmacological effect. Only the free drug molecules can cause an effect. As free molecules leave the circulation, drug molecules are released from plasma protein to re-establish a ratio between the bound and the free molecules. Binding tends to be non-specific and competitive. This means that plasma proteins will bind with many different drugs and these drugs will compete for binding sites on the plasma proteins. Displacement of one drug by another drug may have serious consequences. For example, warfarin can be displaced by tolbutamide producing a risk of haemorrhage, whilst tolbutamide can be displaced by salicylates producing a risk of hypoglycaemia.

- *Placental barrier* – The chorionic villi enclose the foetal capillaries. These are separated from the maternal capillaries by a layer of trophoblastic cells. This barrier will permit the passage of lipid-soluble, non-ionised compounds from mother to foetus but prevents entrance of those substances that are poorly lipid-soluble.

- *Blood-brain barrier* – Capillaries of the central nervous system differ from those in most other parts of the body. They lack channels between endothelial cells through which substances in the blood normally gain access to the extracellular fluid. This barrier constrains the passage of substances from the blood to the brain and cerebrospinal fluid. Lipid-soluble drugs, e.g. diazepam, will pass fairly readily into the central nervous system, where as lipid-insoluble drugs will have little or no effect.

- *Storage sites* – Fat tissue will act as a storage site for lipid-soluble drugs, e.g. anticoagulants. Drugs that have accumulated there, may remain for some time, not being released until after administration of the drugs has ceased. Calcium-containing structures such as bone and teeth can accumulate drugs that are bound to calcium (e.g. tetracycline).

Drug metabolism

Drug metabolism or *biotransformation* refers to the process of modifying or altering the chemical composition of the drug. The pharmacological activity of the drug is usually removed. Metabolites (products of metabolism) are produced which are more polar and less lipid-soluble than the original drug, which ultimately promotes their excretion from the body. Most drug metabolism occurs in the liver, where hepatic enzymes catalyse various biochemical reactions. Metabolism of drugs may also occur in the kidneys, intestinal mucosa, lungs, plasma, and placenta.

Metabolism proceeds in two phases:

- Phase I – These reactions attempt to biotransform the drug to a more polar metabolite. The most common reactions are oxidations, catalysed by mixed function oxidase enzymes. Other phase I reactions include reduction and hydrolysis reactions.

- Phase II – Drugs or phase I metabolites which are not sufficiently polar for excretion by the kidneys, are made more hydrophilic ('water-liking') by conjugation (synthetic) reactions with endogenous compounds provided by the liver. The resulting conjugates are then readily excreted by the kidneys.

With some drugs, if given repeatedly, metabolism of the drugs becomes more effective due to enzyme induction. Therefore larger and larger doses of the drug become required in order to produce the same effect. This is referred to as *drug tolerance*. Tolerance may also develop as a result of adaptive changes at cell receptors.

Various factors affect a patient's ability to metabolise drugs. These include:

- *Genetic differences* – The enzyme systems which control drug metabolism are genetically determined. Some individuals show exaggerated and prolonged responses to drugs such as propranolol which undergo extensive hepatic metabolism.

- *Age* – In the elderly, first pass metabolism may be reduced, resulting in increased bioavailability. In addition, the delayed production and elimination of active metabolites may prolong drug action. Reduced doses may, therefore, be necessary in the elderly. The enzyme systems responsible for conjugation are not fully effective in the neonate and this group of patients may be at an increased risk of toxic effects of drugs.

- *Disease processes* – Liver disease (acute or chronic) will affect metabolism if there is destruction of hepatocytes. Reduced hepatic blood flow as a result of cardiac failure or shock may also reduce the rate of metabolism of drugs.

Drug excretion

Kidneys

Most drugs and metabolites are excreted by the kidneys. Small drug or metabolite molecules may be transported by glomerular filtration into the tubule. This, however, only applies to free drugs and not drugs bound to plasma proteins. Active secretion of some drugs into the lumen of the nephron will also occur. This process however, requires membrane carriers and energy.

Several factors may affect the rate at which a drug is excreted by the kidneys. These include:

- Presence of kidney disease (e.g. renal failure)
- Altered renal blood flow
- pH of urine
- Concentration of the drug in plasma
- Molecular weight of the drug

Bile

Several drugs and metabolites are secreted by the liver into bile. These then enter the first part of the small intestine (the duodenum) via the common bile duct, and continue onwards through the small intestine. Some drugs will be reabsorbed back into the bloodstream from the terminal ileum, and return to the liver by the enterohepatic circulation (Figure 1.1). The drug then undergoes further metabolism or is secreted back into bile. This is referred to as enterohepatic cycling and may extend the duration of action of a drug. Drugs secreted into bile, will ultimately pass through the large intestine and be excreted in faeces.

Figure 1.1 – The enterohepatic circulation

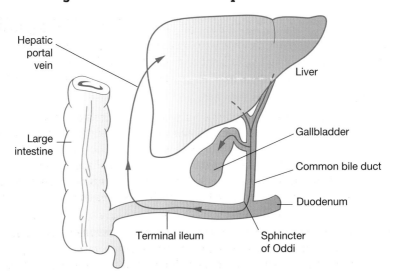

Lungs

Anaesthetic gases and small amounts of alcohol undergo pulmonary excretion.

Breast milk

Milk-producing glands are surrounded by a network of capillaries, and drugs may pass from maternal blood into the breast milk. The amounts of drug may be very small, but may affect a suckling infant who has less ability to metabolise and excrete drugs.

Perspiration, saliva, and tears

Drugs may be excreted passively via these body secretions if the drugs are lipid-soluble.

The processes of drug metabolism and drug excretion will ultimately determine the drug's *half-life*. This is the time taken for the concentration of drug in the blood to fall by half (50%) its original value. Standard dosage intervals are based on half-life calculations. This helps in the setting up of a dosage regime which produces stable plasma drug concentrations, keeping the concentration of drug below toxic levels but above the minimum effective level.

There are occasions when an effective plasma concentration of drug must be reached quickly. This requires a dose of the drug which is larger than is normally given. This is called a *loading dose*. Once the required plasma concentration of drug has been reached, the normal recommended dose is given. This is then continued at regular intervals to maintain a stable plasma concentration and is called the *maintenance dose*. Digoxin may be prescribed in this manner.

Determining plasma concentrations of a drug at frequent intervals is undertaken when patients are prescribed drugs with a narrow *therapeutic index,* e.g. digoxin and lithium. The therapeutic index is the ratio of the drug's toxic dose to its minimally effective dose. Monitoring plasma concentrations can also be used to assess a patient's compliance to drug therapy.

Pharmacodynamics

Whilst pharmacokinetics considers the way in which the body affects a drug by the processes of absorption, distribution, metabolism, and excretion, pharmacodynamics considers the effects of the drug on the body and the mode of drug action.

All body functions are mediated by control systems which depend on enzymes, receptors on cell surfaces, carrier molecules, and specific macromolecules, e.g. DNA. Most drugs act by interfering with these control systems at a molecular level. In order to have their effect, drugs must reach cells via the processes of absorption and distribution already described. Once at their site of action, drugs may work in a very specific manner or non-specifically. Specific mechanisms will be considered first of all.

- *Interaction with receptors on the cell membrane* – A receptor is usually a protein molecule found on the surface of the cell or located intracellularly in the cytoplasm. Drugs frequently interact with receptors to form a drug-receptor complex. In order for a drug to interact with a receptor, it has to

13

Figure 1.2 – Drug-receptor complex

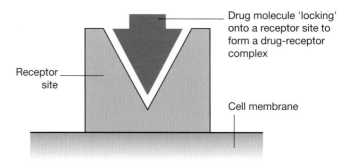

Drug molecule 'locking' onto a receptor site to form a drug-receptor complex

Receptor site

Cell membrane

have a complementary structure in the same way that a key has a structure complementary to the lock in which it fits (Figure 1.2). Very few drugs are truly specific to a particular receptor and some drugs will combine with more than one type of receptor. However, many drugs show selective activity on one particular receptor-type.

A drug that has an affinity for a receptor, and that once bound to the receptor can cause a specific response, is called an *agonist*. Morphine is an opioid agonist that binds to mu receptors in the central nervous system to depress the appreciation of pain. Drugs that bind to receptors and do not cause a response are called *antagonists* or receptor blockers. These will reduce the likelihood of another drug or chemical binding and hence will reduce or block further drug activity. Antagonists may be *competitive*, in which case they compete with an agonist for receptor sites and inhibit the action of the agonist. The action of the drug depends on whether it is the agonist or antagonist that occupies the most receptors. For example, naloxone is a competitive antagonist for mu receptors and is may be used to treat opioid overdose. It will compete with morphine for mu receptors and reverse the effects of an excessive dose of morphine. A *non-competitive* antagonist will inactivate a receptor so that an agonist cannot have an effect.

Drug-receptor binding is reversible and the response to the drug is gradually reduced once the drug leaves the receptor site.

- *Interference with ion passage through the cell membrane* – Ion channels are selective pores in the cell membrane that allow the movement of ions in and out of the cell. Some drugs will block these channels, which ultimately interferes with ion transport and causes an altered physiological response. Drugs working in this way include nifedipine, verapamil, and lignocaine.

- *Enzyme inhibition or stimulation* – Enzymes are proteins and biological catalysts which speed up the rate of chemical reactions. Some drugs interact with enzymes in a manner similar to the drug-receptor complex mechanism already described. Drugs often resemble a natural substrate and compete with the natural substrate for the enzyme. Drugs interacting with enzymes include aspirin, methotrexate, and angiotensin-converting enzyme (ACE) inhibitors such as enalapril.

- *Incorporation into macromolecules* – Some drugs may be taken up by a larger molecule and will interfere with the normal function of that molecule. For example, when the anticancer drug 5-fluorouracil is incorporated into messenger RNA, taking the place of the molecule uracil, transcription is affected.
- *Interference with metabolic processes of micro-organisms* – Some drugs interfere with metabolic processes that are very specific or unique to micro-organisms and thus kill or inhibit activity of the micro-organism. Penicillin disrupts bacterial cell wall formation whilst trimethroprim inhibits bacterial folic acid synthesis.

Non-specific mechanisms involve:

- *Chemical alteration of the cellular environment* – Drugs may not alter specific cell function, but because they alter the chemical environment around the cell, cellular responses or changes occur. Drugs which have this effect include osmotic diuretics (e.g. mannitol) osmotic laxatives (e.g. lactulose) and antacids (e.g. magnesium hydroxide).
- *Physical alteration of the cellular environment* – Drugs may not alter specific cell function, but because they alter the physical as opposed to the chemical environment around the cell, cellular responses or changes occur. Drugs that have this effect would include docusate sodium, which lowers faecal surface tension and many of the barrier preparations available, which protect the skin.

Undesirable Responses to Drug Therapy

Most drugs are not entirely free of unwanted effects. However, drugs which are frequently prescribed, highly potent, or that have a narrow therapeutic index, are likely to increase the risk of unwanted effects.

Terms used to describe undesirable responses to drugs include:

- *Adverse reaction* – This refers to any undesirable drug effect.
- *Side-effect* – This is used interchangeably with the term adverse reaction. It refers to unwanted but predictable responses to a drug.
- *Toxic effect* – This usually occurs when too much drug has accumulated in the patient. It may be due to an acute high dose of a drug, chronic build up over time or increased sensitivity to the standard dose of a drug.
- *Drug allergy (hypersensitivity)* – The body sees the drug as an antigen and an immune response is established against the drug. This may be an immediate response or delayed.

Factors affecting a patient's response to a drug

Many individual factors will determine an individual's clinical response to a drug. Some of these have already been identified but additional factors will also be considered here. The nurse prescriber should be fully aware of these factors and they should be incorporated into the patient assessment before decisions are made about which drug to prescribe. In addition, they should be considered when monitoring drugs which are already being used by the patient, whether the drugs are prescribed or obtained 'over-the-counter'.

- *Age* – The very young and the elderly particularly have problems related to their ability to metabolise and excrete drugs. Neonatal hepatic enzyme systems are not fully effective, so drug metabolism will be reduced and there is an increased risk of toxicity. In the elderly, delayed metabolism by the liver and a decline in renal function means delayed excretion by the kidneys and drug action may be prolonged. Complicated drug regimes may be difficult for the elderly to follow which may mean inadequate or excessive doses of drugs are consumed.

- *Body weight* – The size of an individual will affect the amount of a drug that is distributed and available to act. The larger the individual, the larger the area for drug distribution. Lipid-soluble drugs may be sequestered in fat stores and not available for use. This is the reason that some drugs are given according to the patient's body weight i.e. *x* milligrams per kilogram of body weight. All patients should have their weight recorded and this should be reassessed regularly if the patient is receiving long term drug treatment.

- *Pregnancy and lactation* – Lipid-soluble, unionised drugs in the free state will cross the placenta (e.g. opiates, warfarin). Some may be teratogenic and cause foetal malformation. Drugs can also be transferred to the suckling infant via breast milk and have adverse effects on the child (e.g. sedatives, anticonvulsants, and caffeine). A full drug history should be obtained pre-conception where possible or as soon as pregnancy has been diagnosed. Women must be educated not to take medication without consulting a physician, pharmacist, midwife or nurse.

- *Nutritional status* – Patients who are malnourished may have altered drug distribution and metabolism. Inadequate dietary protein may affect enzyme activity and slow the metabolism of drugs. A reduction in plasma protein levels may mean that more free drug is available for activity. A loss of body fat stores will mean less sequestering of the drug in fat and more drug available for activity. Normal doses in the severely malnourished may lead to toxicity. Nutritional assessment of patients is, therefore, essential and malnutrition should be managed accordingly.

- *Food-drug interactions* – The presence of food may enhance or inhibit the absorption of a drug. For example, orange juice (vitamin C) will enhance the absorption of iron sulphate, but dairy produce reduces the absorption of tetracycline. Monoamine oxidase inhibitors must not be taken with foods rich in tyramine, such as cheese, meat yeast extracts, some types of alcoholic drinks, and other products, due to toxic effects occurring, such as a sudden hypertensive crisis. Nurses should have some knowledge of common food-drug interactions and drug administration may need timing in relation to mealtimes.

- *Disease processes* – Altered functioning of many body systems will affect a patient's response to a drug. Only a few examples are therefore given.

Changes in gut motility and therefore transit time may affect absorption rates (e.g. with diarrhoea and vomiting, absorption is reduced). Loss of absorptive surface in the small intestine, as occurs in Crohn's disease will affect absorption.

Hepatic disease – (e.g. hepatitis, cirrhosis, and liver failure) will reduce metabolism of drugs and lead to a gradual accumulation of drugs and risk of toxicity.

Renal disease – (e.g. acute and chronic renal failure) will reduce excretion of drugs and drugs may accumulate.

Circulatory diseases – (e.g. heart failure and peripheral vascular disease) will reduce distribution and transport of drugs.

- *Mental and emotional factors* – Many factors may affect a patient's ability to comply with their drug regime. These include confusion, amnesia, identified mental illness, stress, bereavement and many others. These types of problems may lead to inadequate or excessive use of medication resulting in unsuccessful treatment or serious adverse effects. The nurse must consider these issues in the patient assessment.

- *Genetic and ethnic factors* – Enzyme systems controlling drug metabolism are genetically determined and therefore, genetic variation leads to differences in patients' abilities to metabolise drugs. For example, some individuals possess an atypical form of the enzyme pseudocholinesterase. When these individuals are given the muscle relaxant suxamethonium, prolonged paralysis occurs and recovery from the drug takes longer. Different races of people are also known to dispose of drugs at different rates.

Further Reading

Baer CL, Williams BR (1996). *Clinical Pharmacology and Nursing* (3rd edn). Springhouse, PA: Springhouse Corporation.
Clarke JB, Queener SF, Karb V (1997). *Pharmacologic Basis of Nursing Practice* (5th edn). St Louis: Mosby.
Downie G, Mackenzie J (1999). *Pharmacology and Drug Management for Nurses* (2nd edn). Edinburgh: Churchill Livingstone.
Galbraith A, Bullock S, Manias E, Richards A, Hunt B (1999). *Fundamentals of Pharmacology: A Text for Nurses and Health Professionals*. Singapore: Addison Wesley Longman.
Pinnell NL (1996). *Nursing Pharmacology*. Philadelphia: W.B. Saunders.
Rang HP, Dale MM, Ritter JM (1999). *Pharmacology* (4th edn). Edinburgh: Churchill Livingstone.
Springhouse (2001). *Clinical Pharmacology Made Incredibly Easy!* Springhouse, PA: Springhouse Corporation.
Trounce JR, Gould D (2000). *Clinical Pharmacology for Nurses* (16th edn). Edinburgh: Churchill Livingstone.

Chapter 2

Preparations for the Prevention and Treatment of Infection

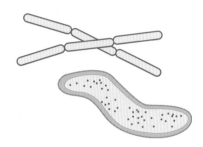

In this chapter two main groups of drugs will be considered. Firstly, drugs that contribute to the prevention of infection will be dealt with. These are immunomodulating agents or vaccines, which stimulate the immune system and enhance immune protection. Secondly, the chapter deals with the different groups of antibacterials that are available to the nurse prescriber, when required to treat established infection.

The Immune Response

In order for the nurse prescriber to fully understand the nature of vaccines and the vaccination process, an appreciation of the human immune response is required.

Specific immunity

Specific immunity is provided by the co-ordinated activities of T and B cells (lymphocytes). These cell types respond to the presence of specific antigens. Antigens are any substances that induce an immune response, and include proteins, carbohydrates, and lipids associated with invading organisms. The T cells are responsible for cell-mediated immunity or defence against abnormal cells and pathogens inside cells. The B cells however, provide humoral immunity (antibody-mediated immunity) or defence against antigens and pathogens in body fluids.

Humoral immunity

In humoral immunity, there are three key phases to the process. These are

- recognition
- attack
- memory

In recognition, B cells recognise an antigen and divide to form an army of identical cells. The daughter cells form plasma cells that synthesise antibodies specific to the antigen. In attack, the plasma cells release their antibodies, which bind on to the antigen to make it harmless and label it for destruction by other agents. In the memory stage, B cells differentiate into memory cells, which will protect against exposure to the same antigen at some point in the future.

Cell-mediated immunity

Like humoral immunity, the same three key phases are also present in cell-mediated immunity.

During the recognition phase, the antigen has to be presented to the T cells. The T cells must then be activated by exposure to an antigen. An activated T cell enlarges, multiplies and forms an army of identical T cells.

In the attack phase, different types of T cells play different roles. Helper T cells play a central coordinating role in both humoral and cellular immunity. Cytotoxic T cells are able to directly attack and kill various different cells. As the pathogen is destroyed, suppressor T cells release lymphokines that inhibit T and B cell activity. This slows down the immune reaction and prevents it from getting out of control.

As the helper T cells recruit more and more cells during the attack phase, the immune system becomes an overwhelming force for the pathogen. Some of the T cells become memory cells and will be responsible for mounting a rapid attack should the same pathogen be encountered later in life (Saladin, 2001).

Forms of Immunity

Innate immunity is present at birth, genetically determined, and there is no relationship to previous exposure to antigens. Acquired immunity is not present at birth and it only occurs after exposure to a specific antigen. Acquired immunity can be active or passive.

Active immunity appears following exposure to an antigen, and can result from natural exposure to an antigen in the environment (called natural acquired immunity) or from deliberate exposure to an antigen (called induced active immunity). Induced active immunity will stimulate antibody production under controlled conditions and means that the body will be able to overcome natural exposure to the pathogen in the future. This is the basic principle behind vaccination or immunisation.

Passive immunity arises following the transfer of antibodies from another person. Natural passive immunity occurs when a mother transfers antibodies to her baby either via the placenta during pregnancy, or via breast milk when feeding her child. Induced passive immunity involves administering antibodies (in the form of antisera) to prevent disease or fight infection (Martini, 2001).

Responses to antigen exposure

The first exposure to an antigen is called the primary response. If an individual is exposed to the same antigen again, it triggers a secondary response. Primary and secondary responses are characteristic of both cell-mediated immunity and humoral immunity.

The primary response

The primary response does not appear immediately as the antigen has to activate B cells which must then differentiate into plasma cells. During this response the level of antibody activity in the plasma does not reach a peak until 1–2 weeks after the initial exposure. The two types of antibodies involved in the primary response are immunoglobulin M (IgM) and immunoglobulin G (IgG). IgM appears first in the plasma, being secreted from the plasma cells, and it provides an immediate but quite limited defence against the pathogen. Levels of IgG rise more slowly as the stimulated B cells are generating large numbers of memory cells as well as plasma cells. However, large quantities of IgG can be produced to fight the infection.

The secondary response

If the body is exposed to an antigen for the second time, memory B cells respond immediately and faster than the B cells that were stimulated on the first exposure. This is due to the fact that memory B cells are activated at lower antigen concentrations and also because they produce more effective and destructive antibodies (Martini, 2001). Antibodies are secreted in huge quantities, to what is known as the secondary response to antigen exposure. Plasma antibody levels increase very rapidly and reach much higher levels than during the primary response (Figure 2.1).

The speed of the primary response and the low levels of antibodies produced may not prevent an infection, however the rapid secondary response is likely to be very effective. The effectiveness of the secondary response is one of the main principles behind using vaccination to prevent infectious disease.

Figure 2.1 – Primary and secondary responses

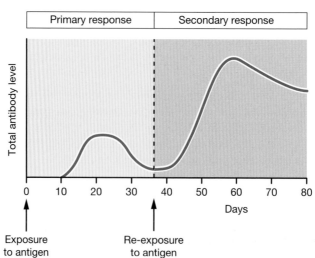

Prevention of Infectious Diseases

Several vaccines are available for those nurse prescribers involved in vaccination of patients. Nurses must however, have received training and be competent in all aspects of immunisation, including the contraindications to specific vaccines. Adequate training must have been given in the recognition and management of anaphylaxis (DoH, 1996).

Preparations for the prevention of infection:

- Tuberculin PPD
- Vaccine, Adsorbed Diptheria
- Vaccine, Adsorbed Diptheria for adults and adolescents
- Vaccine, Adsorbed Diptheria and Tetanus
- Vaccine, Adsorbed Diptheria and Tetanus for adults and adolescents
- Vaccine, Adsorbed Diptheria, Tetanus and Pertussis
- Vaccine, BCG
- Vaccine, BCG percutaneous
- Vaccine, Diptheria Toxoid, Tetanus Toxoid, and Acellular Pertussis
- Vaccine, Haemophilus Influenzae Type B (Hib)
- Vaccine, Haemophilus Influenzae Type B (Hib) with Diptheria, Tetanus and Pertussis
- Vaccine, Haemophilus Influenzae Type B, Diptheria, Tetanus and Pertussis
- Vaccine, Hepatitis A injection
- Vaccine, Hepatitis A with Typhoid
- Vaccine, Hepatitis A, Inactivated, with Recombinant (DNA) Hepatitis B
- Vaccine, Hepatitis B
- Vaccine, Influenza
- Vaccine, Live Measles, Mumps and Rubella
- Vaccine, Meningococcal Group C Conjugate
- Vaccine, Meningococcal Polysaccharide A and C
- Vaccine, Pneumococcal
- Vaccine, Poliomyelitis, Inactivated
- Vaccine, Poliomyelitis, Live (oral)
- Vaccine, Rubella, Live
- Vaccine, Tetanus, Adsorbed
- Vaccine, Typhoid, Live Attenuated (oral)
- Vaccine, Typhoid, Polysaccharide

All vaccines listed are administered by injection except for the live poliomyelitis vaccine, and live attenuated typhoid vaccine, which are administered by mouth.

Mode of action

In active immunisation or vaccination, a primary response to a particular pathogen is intentionally stimulated. This sensitises immune cells for a potential subsequent exposure to the pathogen. Upon re-exposure to the pathogen at a later date, the memory of the previous encounter triggers a much quicker immune response or secondary response.

In order to stimulate the primary immune response, the vaccine must be able to target the immune system appropriately, i.e. cellular and/or humoral mechanisms. Most vaccines consist of either, attenuated organisms, killed organisms, inactivated toxins, or subcellular fragments and more recently genes for antigens in viral 'vectors', and DNA itself (Lydyard *et al.*, 2000).

The vaccine types for those vaccines available to the nurse prescriber, are given in Table 2.1.

Wood (2001) identifies the major types of vaccines in current use:

- *Killed or inactivated organisms* – This involves treating an organism with heat or chemicals so that it is no longer infectious. These vaccines stimulate good antibody responses but not cell-mediated immunity.

- *Attenuated organisms* – These pathogens are still viable and cause infection but not disease. They stimulate cell-mediated immunity as well as humoral immunity.

Table 2.1 – Common vaccines

Organism	Vaccine type
Bacterial infection	
Diptheria	Toxoid
Tetanus	Toxoid
Pertussis (whooping cough)	Killed bacteria
Meningitis – *Neissera meningitides*	Capsular polysaccharide
Streptococcus pneumoniae	Capsular polysaccharide
Typhoid	Live, attenuated
	Capsular polysaccharide
Tuberculosis	Live, attenuated
Viral infection	
Influenza	Inactivated virus
Hepatitis (A and B)	Inactivated virus
	Recombinant vaccine
Measles	Attenuated virus
Mumps	Attenuated virus
Rubella	Attenuated virus
Poliomyelitis	Live, attenuated virus

- *Subunit vaccines* – An antibody response against a specific component of the organism is sometimes sufficient to provide immunity. Many bacteria have a polysaccharide coat which when incorporated into a vaccine induces enough antibody to provide immunity. Subunit vaccines can also be proteins.
- *Toxoids* – Some organisms cause disease solely through toxin production. It is possible to vaccinate against the toxin. The toxin is treated chemically so that its toxicity is lost but it retains its antigenicity.

Contraindications

Most vaccines have some contraindications to their use. They should not be administered during acute illness, in those with some forms of hypersensitivity, to pregnant women, to those with impaired immune response and to patients with some forms of malignancy. The nurse prescriber must consult the individual product literature and the DoH (1996) handbook 'Immunisation against Infectious Disease', before administering vaccines.

Adverse effects

Adverse effects vary from a few symptoms to a mild form of the disease. Fever and malaise may arise, and some individuals may complain of discomfort at the injection site. Anaphylactic reactions are rare but serious when they do occur. The nurse prescriber must consult the individual product literature and the DoH (1996) handbook 'Immunisation against Infectious Disease', to determine the adverse effects for the vaccine administered.

Nursing Points

Recommendations for immunisation reflect the present national immunisation policy and can be found in the DoH (1996) handbook, previously mentioned.

Nurses providing immunisation should have received appropriate training and be proficient in the appropriate techniques. Preparations must be made for the management of anaphylaxis and other immediate reactions.

Treatment of Infection

The NPEF enables the nurse prescriber to select from a range of antibacterials, in order to treat established infection. The specific details regarding the infections to be treated can be found in the relevant, subsequent chapters. Problems and ailments resulting in infection include:

- acne, impetigo
- conjunctivitis
- blepharitis
- otitis externa
- urinary tract infection

Figure 2.2 – Structure of a bacterial cell

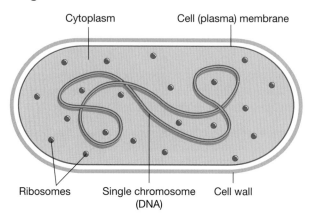

In order to understand how antibacterials have their effect, the nurse prescriber requires knowledge about the structure of a 'generalised' bacterial cell (Figure 2.2).

Surrounding the bacterial cell, is a cell wall containing peptidoglycan. This substance is unique to bacteria and not found in human cells. Within the cell wall is the selectively permeable bacterial cell membrane which is similar to that in the human cell. It consists of a phospholipid bilayer and membrane proteins, but it does not contain sterols. The cytoplasm is found within the cell membrane. As in human cells, the cytoplasm contains soluble proteins (many enzymes), ribosomes for protein synthesis, inorganic ions and intermediary molecules of metabolism. The bacterial cell, unlike the human cell, has no nucleus. The genetic material exists in a single chromosome lying within the cytoplasm.

Antibacterial drugs can be classified in several ways:

- They can be described as being bacteriostatic or bacteriocidal. Bacteriostatic drugs inhibit bacterial growth without killing the cell. The human immune system will ultimately destroy the organism. Bacteriocidal drugs kill the bacteria.
- By chemical structure (see the following list of preparations).
- According to their mode of action (described later in this chapter).
- According to their range or spectrum of activity. They may be 'broad spectrum' or 'narrow spectrum'.

Preparations for the treatment of infection:

Penicillinase-resistant penicillins
- Flucloxacillin

Broad-spectrum penicillins
- Amoxicillin

Tetracyclines
- Tetracycline
- Doxycycline
- Minocycline
- Oxytetracycline

Aminoglycosides
- Gentamycin
- Neomycin

Macrolides
- Erythromycin

Other antibacterials
- Chloramphenicol
- Fusidic acid
- Trimethoprim
- Metronidazole
- Nitrofurantoin
- Clindamycin

The above drugs are available to the nurse prescriber in various forms (oral, eye drops, ear drops, topical), depending on the infection being treated.

Mode of action

There are five major mechanisms by which antibacterial drugs have their effect. These are
- inhibition of synthesis and damage to the bacterial cell wall
- inhibition of synthesis and damage to the bacterial cell membrane
- modification of bacterial nucleic acid synthesis
- inhibition or modification of bacterial protein synthesis
- modification of bacterial energy metabolism

(Wingard *et al.*, 1991)

Inhibition of synthesis and damage to the bacterial cell wall

Penicillins, penicillinase-resistant penicillins, broad-spectrum penicillins, and cephalosporins all disrupt formation of the peptidoglycan layer of the cell wall. The bacterial cell is then unable to maintain its osmotic gradient and begins to swell. Eventually the cell ruptures and dies.

Inhibition of synthesis and damage to the bacterial cell membrane

Polymyxins bind to membrane phospholipids and alter permeability to sodium and potassium ions. Holes are generated in the membrane and this disrupts the cell's osmotic gradient. The cell eventually ruptures.

Modification of bacterial nucleic acid synthesis

Quinolones inhibit replication of bacterial deoxyribonucleic acid (DNA). They block the activity of DNA gyrase, an enzyme essential for DNA replication and repair. Metronidazole acts via an intermediate which inhibits the synthesis of bacterial DNA and breaks down existing DNA.

The precise action of nitrofurantoin is not established. It is thought that the drug is reduced to an unstable metabolite which causes DNA strand breakage and bacterial damage.

Inhibition or modification of bacterial protein synthesis

Several groups of antibacterials prevent the production of essential bacterial cell proteins. Tetracyclines, aminoglycosides, macrolides, clindamycin, and chloramphenicol all act by binding to one of the subunits of the bacterial ribosomes where proteins are actually manufactured, and hence prevent protein synthesis. Fusidic acid prevents transfer ribonucleic acid (tRNA) binding to the ribosomes. Protein synthesis inhibitors tend to have bacteriostatic properties.

Modification of bacterial energy metabolism

Trimethoprim acts by inhibition of the folate pathway in bacteria. Bacteria have to synthesise their own folate derivatives which are important in intracellular reactions. Trimethoprim interrupts the conversion of dihydrofolic acid to tetrahydrofolic acid, by inhibiting the enzyme dihydrofolate reductase.

Contraindications

Penicillins
- Penicillin hypersensitivity.

Tetracyclines
- Renal impairment, pregnancy, and breast feeding, children under 12 years.

Aminoglycosides
- Myasthenia gravis, hypersensitivity.

Macrolides
- Hypersensitivity. Estolate contraindicated in hepatic disease.

Chloramphenicol
- Pregnancy and breast feeding, porphyria.

Fusidic acid
- Hypersensitivity.

Trimethoprim

- Renal impairment and blood dyscrasias.

Metronidazole

- Hypersensitivity, hepatic impairment.

Nitrofurantoin

- G6PD deficiency, impaired renal function in infants under 3 months.

Clindamycin

- Diarrhoeal states.

Adverse effects

- Penicillins and penicillinase-resistant penicillins

Oral preparations of flucloxacillin may cause hypersensitivity reactions (urticaria, fever, joint pains, rashes, angioedema, and anaphylaxis), haemolytic anaemia, interstitial nephritis, thrombocytopenia, neutropenia, paraesthesia, diarrhoea, and antibiotic-associated colitis.

- Broad-spectrum penicillins

Oral preparations of amoxicillin may cause nausea, vomiting, diarrhoea, rashes, hypersensitivity reactions (urticaria, fever, joint pains, rashes, angioedema, and anaphylaxis), haemolytic anaemia, interstitial nephritis, thrombocytopenia, neutropenia, and paraesthesia.

- Tetracyclines

Oral preparations of tetracycline, doxycycline, minocycline, and oxytetracycline may cause nausea, vomiting, diarrhoea, dysphagia, oesophageal irritation, hypersensitivity (rash, urticaria, angioedema, anaphylaxis, and exfoliative dermatitis), headache, visual disturbance, hepatotoxicity, pancreatitis, photosensitivity, blood dyscrasias, and skin discoloration. Topical tetracycline may cause mild skin irritation and rarely sensitisation.

- Aminoglycosides

Gentamycin and neomycin are included in topical preparations and may cause irritation, burning, stinging, and itching.

- Macrolides

Oral preparations of erythromycin may cause nausea, vomiting, abdominal discomfort, diarrhoea, urticaria, rashes, and other allergic reactions, reversible hearing loss, cholestatic jaundice, and cardiac effects. Topical erythromycin may cause mild irritation of the skin and sensitisation.

- Chloramphenicol

Topical chloramphenicol may cause transient stinging.

- Fusidic acid

Rarely, hypersensitivity to topical administration has been reported.

- Trimethoprim

Oral trimethoprim may cause nausea, vomiting, rashes, pruritus, hyperkalaemia and depression of haematopoiesis, photosensitivity, and allergic reactions (angioedema and anaphylaxis).

- Metronidazole

Oral metronidazole may cause nausea, vomiting, rashes, furred tongue, drowsiness, headache, dizziness, ataxia, urticaria, pruritus, angioedema, anaphylaxis, hepatitis, jaundice, myalgia, joint pains, thrombocytopenia, and aplastic anaemia. Vaginal application of metronidazole gel may cause local irritation, abnormal discharge, candidiasis, and increased pelvic pressure.

- Nitrofurantoin

Oral nitrofurantoin may cause nausea, vomiting, anorexia, diarrhoea, peripheral neuropathy, acute and chronic pulmonary reactions, angioedema, urticaria, rash, pruritus, jaundice, hepatitis, pancreatitis, arthralgia, and blood dyscrasias.

- Clindamycin

Topical clindamycin may cause mild irritation of the skin and sensitisation. Clindamycin vaginal cream may damage latex condoms and diaphragms.

Nursing Points

Before prescribing an antibacterial, the nurse prescriber must consider the following factors related to the patient: previous history of antibacterial therapy, previous history of allergy, present hepatic and renal function, and other previously listed contraindications.

The dose of drug to be prescribed will depend on several factors including age, weight, and renal function.

Local antibacterial policies may indicate which drugs should be prescribed and the nurse prescriber should consult these.

Viral infections should not be treated with antibacterials.

The nurse prescriber should not be prescribing antibacterials as prophylaxis. Specimens should be obtained from the affected site for culture and sensitivity so that the causative organism can be identified. When the organism has been isolated, treatment may be changed to another drug if deemed more appropriate.

Some oral antibacterials should be administered at specific times:

- Amoxicillin is not affected by gastric acid and can be taken without concern about meals.
- Tetracycline should be administered on an empty stomach. It should be taken 1 h before meals or 2 h after. Antidiarrhoeals, antacids and dairy

products will adversely affect absorption. Doxycycline and minocycline can be taken on a full or empty stomach (Galbraith *et al.*, 1999). All tetracyclines should be swallowed whole while sitting or standing.

- Nitrofurantoin should be taken after meals to avoid gastric irritation.

The patient should receive education about timing and spacing of medication, adverse effects and the importance of completing the prescribed course.

If allergic reactions occur, the drug should be discontinued and a physician notified immediately.

References

Department of Health (1996). *Immunisation Against Infectious Disease*. London: The Stationery Office.

Galbraith A, Bullock S, Manias E, Richards A, Hunt B (1999). *Fundamentals of Pharmacology: A Text for Nurses and Health Professionals*. Singapore: Addison Wesley Longman.

Lydyard PM, Whelan A, Fanger MW (2000). *Instant Notes in Immunology*. Oxford: BIOS.

Martini FH (2001). *Fundamentals of Anatomy and Physiology* (5th edn). Upper Saddle River: Prentice Hall.

Saladin KS (2001). *Anatomy and Physiology: The Unity of Form and Function* (2nd edn). Boston: McGraw Hill.

Wingard LB, Brody TM, Larner J, Schwartz A (1991). *Human Pharmacology: Molecular to Clinical*. St Louis: Mosby Year Book.

Wood P (2001). *Understanding Immunology*. Harlow: Prentice Hall.

Nociceptors are abundant in the superficial portions of the skin, joint capsules, within the periostea of bones, and around the walls of blood vessels. However, there are very few of these receptors in deep tissue or visceral organs.

Several different types of nociceptors exist. These include:

- Those sensitive to extremes in temperature
- Those sensitive to mechanical damage
- Those sensitive to dissolved chemicals, such as those released by injured cells

Stimuli that are very powerful will excite all three types of receptors. Painful sensations are therefore sometimes described in very similar terms.

When tissue damage occurs, two different types of pain can be distinguished. The sharp localised pain felt at the time of the injury and the longer lasting discomfort felt shortly afterwards. These two different types of sensations are sometimes referred to as fast and slow pain. Their differences are due to the different types of receptors stimulated, the route travelled by the impulse, and its destinations within the nervous system (Rutishauser, 1994).

During tissue injury, damage to the cell membrane occurs. The injured cell membrane releases a substance called arachidonic acid into the interstitial fluid. Within the interstitial fluid, the enzyme cyclo-oxygenase converts arachidonic acid into prostaglandins of differing types which may have varying effects (Martini, 2001).

Prostaglandins are very powerful substances, which act locally to co-ordinate cellular activity. They are effective in minute quantities and almost all tissues in the body respond to, and release, these substances (Martini, 2001). The effects of prostaglandins vary depending on their nature and where they are released. When released in response to tissue damage, they stimulate nociceptors in the surrounding area.

Preparations available to the nurse prescriber for the management of pain are considered under the following headings:

- Analgesia for general use
- Non-steroidal anti-inflammatory drugs (NSAIDs)

Analgesics for General Use

Preparations for pain management:

- Aspirin tablets and suppositories
- Codeine phosphate tablets
- Dihydrocodeine continus (DHC Continus®)
- Dihydrocodeine forte tablets (DF118 Forte®) } *See* information about Schedule drugs on page 30
- Dihydrocodeine tablets
- Nefopam hydrochloride tablets (Acupan®)
- Paracetamol preparations

Aspirin

Aspirin (acetylsalicylic acid) is a non-steroidal anti-inflammatory drug (NSAID), with duration of action of approximately 4 h. This preparation is primarily used to treat mild and moderate pain arising from a number of causes including dysmenorrhoea and headaches. Aspirin is particularly advantageous in rheumatic and osteoarthritis conditions, where its anti-inflammatory properties are especially helpful. Its antipyretic action is also very effective in individuals suffering from colds and influenza who have a raised body temperature.

Dosage

Adults and children over 12 years, routine dose 300 mg to 600 mg (1–2 tablets) every 4–6 h for mild to moderate pain and pyrexia. Do not exceed 2.4 g daily without seeking advice from a doctor.

Mode of action

As outlined earlier in the chapter, prostaglandins act as chemical messengers released to co-ordinate local cellular activity. Prostaglandins, formed by most cells of the body, and released in response to a number of stimuli, are major contributors to inflammation and pain. Aspirin acts by suppressing the formation of prostaglandins. Aspirin and other NSAIDs act by blocking the enzyme cyclo-oxygenase, responsible for converting arachidonic acid (a fatty acid released from cell membranes following injury), into prostaglandins (Figure 3.2). The analgesic action of these preparations are therefore largely local, peripherally acting in damaged tissue, rather than centrally in the brain.

Figure 3.2 – The action of aspirin and other NSAIDs

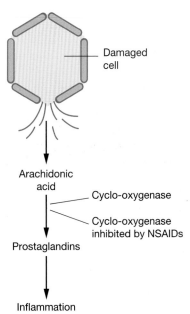

The antipyretic activity of aspirin is also explained by prostaglandin inhibition. When an individual is suffering from a fever, prostaglandins are released in the brain where they have a powerful pyrogenic effect, resetting the hypothalamus or temperature-regulating centre of the brain at a higher level. Aspirin enables this centre to be reset at the normal level (Trounce, 1994).

Adverse effects and contraindications

Aspirin has a number of adverse effects and is contraindicated in several groups of patients. Each of these is outlined below:

- *Gastric irritation and bleeding*

Aspirin can irritate the gastric mucosal lining causing epigastric distress, nausea, and vomiting. It may also cause gastric ulceration, bleeding, exacerbation of peptic ulcer symptoms, and erosive gastritis. These symptoms are due, in part, to aspirin inhibiting the production of prostaglandins in the gastric mucosa. This leads to a reduction in the production of mucus secretion, which increases the likelihood of gastric mucosal damage. If bleeding occurs, blood loss can be as much as 10 ml to 30 ml daily and anaemia may develop if the drug is taken continuously over a long duration. The adverse effects of aspirin can be reduced if it is taken with food, or in its soluble form. However, aspirin should be avoided in patients with a history of gastric problems.

- *Anticoagulation*

During tissue injury, blood vessels become damaged. Within seconds, platelets arrive at the site of the injury and adhere to the damaged vessel (platelet adhesion), and also to each other (platelet aggregation), to form a platelet plug. Arachidonic acid, released from cell membranes following tissue injury, plays an important part in platelet aggregation. Aspirin intervenes in the synthesis of Thromboxane A_2 by inhibiting the enzyme cyclo-oxygenase, and inhibits platelet aggregation. This gives rise to an overall anticoagulation effect (Nathan, 1995). Furthermore, if aspirin is given in large doses it interferes with the body's clotting mechanism and prolongs bleeding time. It should not be prescribed for patients suffering from haemophilia.

- *Hypersensitivity*

Individuals suffering from asthma or allergic conditions are more likely to suffer from hypersensitivity to aspirin. As many as one in ten patients suffering from asthma may be hypersensitive to this preparation (Nathan, 1995). Therefore, unless aspirin has been taken previously without problems, it should be avoided in asthmatics and in patients sensitive to the drug or other NSAIDs.

- *Renal and hepatic disease*

Aspirin can cause liver and kidney impairment. Therefore, patients with renal or hepatic disease should avoid aspirin.

- *Pregnancy*

If aspirin is taken during the third trimester of pregnancy, it can give rise to a number of problems. These include: an adverse effect on the development of the foetus, prolonged pregnancy and labour, and increased bleeding before, during, and after delivery (Govoni and Hayes, 1990).

- *Reye's syndrome*

Aspirin should not be given to children under 12 years or breast feeding mothers, as it may cause Reye's syndrome. This syndrome is a disease of childhood in which swelling of the brain and liver inflammation occurs following a viral infection. Viruses include varicella and influenza B. Reye's syndrome is related to the virus, and appears at the time the child is recovering from the infection. However, there is evidence to suggest, that it is also related to aspirin-taking during the viral infection (McCance and Heuther, 1994).

- *Toxicity*

When the daily dosage of aspirin is more than 4 g, toxicity may occur. Tinnitus (ringing in the ears) is the most common effect and this may be accompanied by a degree of reversible hearing loss. Other symptoms associated with toxicity are hyperventilation, respiratory acidosis and fever.

Drug interactions

Aspirin interacts significantly with a number of drugs. These drugs, and the interactive effects produced, are outlined in Table 3.1.

Nursing Points

Aspirin exhibits analgesic, anti-inflammatory, and antipyretic properties and is used for the treatment of mild to moderate pain. Aspirin acts significantly with a number of other drugs (Table 3.1). It also has a number of adverse effects and is contraindicated in patients suffering from gastric problems, asthmatic or allergic conditions, and renal or hepatic problems. It should also be avoided in patients in their third trimester of pregnancy, breastfeeding mothers, and children under 12 years.

Aspirin is occasionally prescribed by doctors for rheumatic conditions. Nurse prescribers should not prescribe aspirin for these conditions. Aspirin may also be prescribed by the doctor in low doses (e.g. 75 mg daily) to prevent the recurrence of cerebrovascular or cardiovascular disease. Nurse prescribers should not prescribe aspirin for this condition. If patients are being treated in this manner, and taking a regular low daily dose of aspirin, they must be cautioned against taking additional aspirin as a routine analgesic.

Codeine phosphate (*see* page 30)

Codeine phosphate is an opioid or narcotic analgesic, which is chemically closely related to morphine but is much less potent. It is therefore used mainly as an oral analgesic for mild to moderate types of pain. Unlike morphine, it causes little or no euphoria, little respiratory depression and is rarely addictive. Codeine is frequently combined with aspirin or paracetamol in preparations, as it potentiates the activity of both. Other uses of codeine are as an antidiarrhoeal and antitussive.

Table 3.1 – Drugs that interact with aspirin and the effect produced

Drug therapy	Interactive effect
Anticoagulants, e.g. warfarin	Increased risk of bleeding due to enhanced antiplatelet effect
Antacids and adsorbents	Increased urine alkalinity Increased excretion of aspirin
Antiepileptics, e.g. phenytoin and valporate	Enhancement of effect of phenytoin and valporate
Corticosteroids, e.g. prednisolone	Increased risk of gastrointestinal bleeding and ulceration
Cytotoxics, i.e. methotrexate	Reduced excretion rate and increased toxicity
Diuretics	Antagonism of diuretic effect of spironolactone; reduced excretion of acetazolamide (risk of toxicity)
Metoclopramide	Metoclopramide enhances effect of aspirin (increased rate of absorption)
Mifepristone	Manufacturer recommends avoid aspirin until 8–12 days after mifepristone administration
Uricosurics	Effects of probenecid and sulphinpyrazone reduced

N.B. Aspirin should not be given with other NSAIDs (because of increased adverse effects)

Mode of action

Opioid or narcotic analgesics are centrally acting drugs that act upon receptors in the central nervous system. They have no anti-inflammatory effects.

There are at least four different opioid receptor-types present in the brain and spinal cord. These receptors, designated a letter of the Greek alphabet, have been located in specific regions of the brain and spinal cord, and are bound by endogenous opioids. These substances are the body's natural painkillers, which bind to the opioid receptors and suppress pain messages from the periphery to the central nervous system.

The mu (μ) receptors are found in the dorsal horn of the spinal cord and thalamus and when acted on by endogenous β-endorphin, produce analgesia, respiratory depression, and euphoria. The kappa (κ) receptors are located in the hypothalamus and when acted on by dynorphin, produce analgesia, sedation, miosis, and hypothermia. Epsilon (ε) receptors in the hippocampus and amygdala are bound by enkephalin and produce some psychotic effects and dysphoria. Delta (δ) receptors in the limbic system produce behavioural changes and hallucinations when acted on by unknown endogenous opioids (Galbraith et al., 1999).

Opioid analgesia such as morphine, codeine, and pethidine are all opioid receptor agonists, which will bind to specific opiate receptors and mimic the activity of the endogenous opiates. This produces important clinical effects such as pain relief and euphoria for some patients, however, there are also some negative, unrequired effects such as respiratory depression and sedation.

Contraindications

Codeine phosphate is a morphine salt, and all morphine salts are contraindicated in acute respiratory depression, severe respiratory disease and hypersensitivity to opioids.

Adverse effects

Drowsiness, sedation, dizziness, lethargy, mood changes, bradycardia, palpitations, hypotension, tachycardia, dry mouth, miosis, nausea, vomiting, constipation, anorexia, urinary retention, flushing, rash, urticaria, sweating, hypothermia, and respiratory depression.

Nursing Points

Pain assessment and evaluation should be undertaken regularly.

The patient should be made aware of the potential adverse effects of the drug. Constipation is a common problem and a high fibre diet should be encouraged. Some patients may require a laxative during the period they are taking codeine.

The patient should avoid driving or other hazardous activities if drowsiness is a problem.

Alcohol and other central nervous system depressants should be avoided.

Dihydrocodeine tartrate (*see* page 30)

Dihydrocodeine is an opioid or narcotic analgesic with an analgesic efficacy similar to that of codeine. It is indicated in moderate to severe pain.

The mode of action, contraindications, adverse effects, and nursing points are the same as that described earlier in this chapter for codeine phosphate.

Nefopam

Nefopam is a centrally acting, non-opioid analgesic, completely unrelated to all others. It may be used in the management of persistent, moderate pain that is unresponsive to other non-opioid analgesics.

Mode of action

This has not been fully established but may involve inhibition at dopamine, serotonin or noradrenaline receptors in the central nervous system.

Contraindications

Not to be prescribed for patients with myocardial infarction or convulsive disorders. Not recommended for use in children.

Adverse effects

Nervousness, insomnia, drowsiness, blurred vision, headache, nausea, dry mouth, vomiting, tachycardia, sweating, urinary retention, and discolouration of the urine (pink).

Nursing Points

Pain assessment and evaluation should be undertaken regularly.

Administer the drug with food to decrease the risk of gastrointestinal symptoms.

Inform the patient of the potential adverse effects and to avoid driving or other hazardous activities if drowsiness is a problem.

Paracetamol

Paracetamol (acetominophen) is an effective analgesic and antipyretic but has little anti-inflammatory activity. Paracetamol is used for the relief of mild to moderate pain, such as headaches, joint and muscle pain, and dysmenorrhoea. It is a good alternative to aspirin. By comparison it is relatively free from adverse effects, although its use is cautioned in patients with hepatic and renal impairment and individuals who suffer from alcohol dependence. It can be used in patients where aspirin has been contraindicated. Therefore, children, the elderly, and pregnant and lactating women may use paracetamol. Furthermore, it has no significant interactions with other drugs. It is also safe to use by patients receiving warfarin, although prolonged regular use of paracetamol may sometimes enhance the anticoagulant effect.

Dosage

The therapeutic dosage of paracetamol for adults is 0.5–1 g every 4–6 h up to a maximum of 4 g daily. This dose is very safe. However, if this dose is exceeded it causes severe hepatotoxicity.

Child 3 months–1 year 60–120 mg; 1–5 years 120–250 mg; 6–12 years 250–500 mg; doses may be repeated every 4–6 h when necessary; maximum of 4 doses in 24 h.

Mode of action

The mechanism by which this preparation works is not fully understood. However, it is thought that paracetamol works by inhibition of cyclo-oxygenase in the central nervous system. There is also evidence to suggest that this compound acts on peripheral pain chemoreceptors (Nathan, 1995).

Metabolism

Paracetamol is absorbed quite rapidly from the gastrointestinal tract and passes to the liver where it is metabolised. It is then transported to the body's tissues in the circulation. During liver metabolism of paracetamol, several metabolites are formed. Acetyl-benzo-quinoneimine is one of these. This is a highly reactive and toxic metabolite which is normally detoxified by conjugation (joining) with glutathione (a protein formed by the liver) and protects the liver from cell damage. However, during an overdose, this detoxification mechanism is overwhelmed.

The amount of quinoneimine formed exceeds the liver's ability to provide enough glutathione. The free toxic metabolite then combines with the cells of the liver causing hepatitis and necrosis, which is often fatal. Toxic levels of paracetamol do not need to be greatly above the therapeutic levels. This makes paracetamol poisoning dangerous, as symptoms of overdose may not appear for two or more days. During this time, overdosage may be accidentally continued. Signs may include, vomiting, jaundice, abdominal tenderness, and hypoglycaemia (Govoni and Hayes, 1990).

It is therefore vitally important that nurses offer suitable advice to patients if prescribing this drug. It needs to be ensured that patients take the correct dose of paracetamol and do not use more than one paracetamol-containing preparation at a time. It is important to encourage the patient to read the labels of all medications carefully. Many over-the-counter-products for pain, sinus problems or colds contain paracetamol alone or in combination with other drugs, including caffeine or aspirin. Acetylcysteine and methionine are effective antidotes for paracetamol poisoning if given within 10–12 h of ingestion.

Nursing Points

Paracetamol exhibits analgesic and antipyretic properties, but has little anti-inflammatory activity. It is used for the treatment of mild to moderate pain. It has few adverse effects and is safe to use in children, the elderly, pregnant and lactating women, and those receiving anticoagulation therapy.

The toxic level of paracetamol is not much greater than the therapeutic level. Cold remedies may contain paracetamol and/or aspirin, and inadvertent overdose is possible. Patients must be warned of this and cautioned not to exceed the recommended dose.

Non-Steroidal Anti-Inflammatory Drugs

Preparations for the management of pain:

- Ibuprofen granules and syrup (Brufen®)
- Ibuprofen modified release tablets and capsules (Brufen Retard®)
- Ibuprofen tablets and suspension

Ibuprofen

Ibuprofen has anti-inflammatory, analgesic and antipyretic properties. It is indicated as an analgesic and anti-inflammatory agent in rheumatic disease (including juvenile arthritis), other musculo-skeletal disorders and soft tissue injuries. It is indicated as an analgesic where there is mild to moderate pain including dysmenorrhoea, post-operative analgesia, migraine, dental problems, fever and pain in children.

Mode of action

Ibuprofen has a mode of action similar to aspirin. The reader should refer to the earlier section about aspirin.

Contraindications

Ibuprofen should be used in caution with the elderly and in people with allergic disorders. Caution should also be taken in patients with renal, cardiac or hepatic impairment.

It is contraindicated in patients with a history of hypersensitivity, hypersensitivity to aspirin or other NSAIDs, asthma, pregnancy, breastfeeding, in coagulation defects and patients with active peptic ulcer disease.

Adverse effects

Gastrointestinal adverse effects include nausea, diarrhoea, bleeding, and ulceration. Hypersensitivity reactions include rashes, angio-oedema, and bronchospasm. Other adverse effects are headache, dizziness, depression, drowsiness, insomnia, vertigo, tinnitus, haematuria, and photosensitivity. Fluid retention and renal failure may occur in those with pre-existing renal problems.

Rare adverse effects include alveolitis, pulmonary eosinophilia, pancreatitis, Stevens–Johnson syndrome, and eye changes.

Nursing Points

The nurse prescriber should assess the patient's medical history with respect to previous gastric bleeding and hypersensitivity. Ibuprofen should not be prescribed in these circumstances. Caution should be taken with patients with cardiac or renal impairment.

Oral medication should be administered with or after food or milk. Sustained-release and enteric coated preparations should be swallowed whole.

The patient should be informed of potential adverse effects and the action to be taken should they occur.

The patient should consult a pharmacist before buying other over-the-counter medications.

Alcohol, aspirin-containing drugs and other NSAIDs should be avoided.

Anxiety in palliative care

Anxiety is defined by Twycross (1997) as a universally unpleasant emotion that can be acute/transient or chronic/persistent. All patients with terminal illness become worried, anxious or frightened at times and such feelings may be recurrent, and are often severe and persistent (WHO, 1998). Symptoms which suggest anxiety include poor concentration, indecisiveness, insomnia, irritability, sweating, tremor, and panic attacks. Twycross (1997) classifies the causes of anxiety in cancer patients as: situational, organic, psychiatric, drug-induced or related to the patient's inner world. It is beyond the scope of this book to consider the management of anxiety in palliative care, however drugs are listed in the extended formulary that can be prescribed by an appropriately trained palliative care nurse, together with the psychological therapy that will be necessary.

Preparations for the management of anxiety:

- Diazepam tablets, oral solution, injection, rectal tubes, and suppositories.
- Lorazepam tablets and injection.

} *See* pages 30 and 31

Mode of action

Diazepam and lorazepam belong to the group of drugs called benzodiazepines. These drugs act on receptors in the central nervous system to potentiate the inhibitory action of gamma-aminobutyric acid (GABA), a natural neurotransmitter (Galbraith *et al.*, 1999). The increased inhibitory neurotransmission produces several potentially useful effects. These include: sedation due to the reduced sensory input to the reticular activating system, a reduction in anxiety (anxiolytic) due to actions on the limbic system and hypothalamus, and anticonvulsant activity (Waller and Renwick, 1994).

Both drugs are for short-term use in anxiety, and diazepam may also be prescribed for skeletal muscle spasm (*see* Chapter 7).

Contraindications

Both drugs are contraindicated in respiratory depression, acute pulmonary insufficiency, sleep apnoea syndrome, and severe hepatic impairment.

Adverse effects

Both drugs may cause daytime drowsiness, confusion, ataxia, amnesia, muscle flaccidity, headache, vertigo, hypotension, gastrointestinal disturbance, tremor, changes in libido, urinary incontinence or retention, blood disorders, and jaundice.

Nursing Points

Therapeutic guidelines for the use of diazepam in palliative care are provided by Twycross (1999), who suggests that the initial dose depends on the patient's previous experience of diazepam or lorazepam, the intensity of the distress and urgency of the relief. Typical doses of diazepam for anxiety management are 2–10 mg orally (as 'immediate' or 'as required' doses) or 2–10 mg orally at night (as an initial daily dose). Rectal diazepam is useful in a crisis or if the patient is moribund. Lorazepam, 1 mg sublingually (equivalent to diazepam 10 mg), can be given as an alternative (Twycross, 1999).

Restlessness and agitation in palliative care

It is beyond the scope of this book to consider the management and treatment of cognitive impairment in the terminally ill. Clients experiencing restlessness, agitation and confusion require assessment, management and evaluation by specially trained nursing and medical staff. The extended formulary however, lists drugs which may be prescribed for restless and agitated patients during the final days of life.

Preparations for the management of restlessness and anxiety:

- Levomepromazine (methotrimeprazine) tablets and injection (Nozinan®)
- Midazolam injection (Hypnovel®) (*see* page 31)

Mode of action

Levomepromazine (Methotrimeprazine) is an antipsychotic (neuroleptic) drug belonging to the group called phenothiazines. Though the exact mechanism of action has still to be determined, levomepromazine antagonises dopamine receptors in the central nervous system, depressing the cerebral cortex, hypothalamus, and limbic system. The clinical effects produced by this action include: a depressant action on conditioned responses and emotional responsiveness; a sedative action useful for the treatment of restlessness and confusion; an anti-emetic effect through blockade of the chemoreceptor trigger zone (CTZ), which is useful to treat vomiting; and antihistamine activity (Waller and Renwick, 1994). The World Health Organisation (1998) suggest this drug is most useful for its sedative effect, in bed-bound patients during the last days of their life.

Midazolam belongs to the benzodiazepine group of drugs, and its mode of action is the same as that described earlier in this chapter for diazepam and lorazepam. It is water-soluble, and is indicated when requiring sedation for terminal agitation.

Contraindications

Levomepromazine (methotrimeprazine) is contraindicated in hypersensitivity, comatose states, central nervous system (CNS) depression, and phaeochromocytoma. It should be avoided in pregnancy.

The contraindications for midazolam are the same as those reported earlier in this chapter for diazepam and lorazepam.

Adverse effects

Adverse effects of levomepromazine (methotrimeprazine) include agranulocytosis, leucopenia, haemolytic anaemia, jaundice, drowsiness, apathy, insomnia, depression, extrapyramidal symptoms, dry mouth, constipation, rashes, nasal congestion, blurred vision, hypotension, tachycardia, and arrhythmias.

The adverse effects for midazolam are the same as those reported earlier in this chapter for diazepam and lorazepam. In addition, respiratory depression and respiratory arrest have been reported.

Nursing Points

Levomepromazine (methotrimeprazine) is administered orally as 12.5–50 mg every 4–8 h, or by subcutaneous infusion at 50–200 mg/24 h.

Midazolam is administered by subcutaneous infusion, at a dose of 20–100 mg/ 24 h.

Neural Tube Defect

Nurse prescribers can play an important role in the health care of women of reproductive age. They can promote the chances of a positive pregnancy outcome by ensuring women are aware of the importance of folic acid supplementation and an adequate dietary intake of folic acid, and should prescribe folic acid to women where appropriate.

Formation of the neural tube

During the third week of development following fertilisation of an ovum, the process of gastrulation occurs. This is the formation of the three primary germ layers (ectoderm, mesoderm, and endoderm) in the developing embryo. Gastrulation provides the basic framework for organogenesis or the formation of organs and organ systems in the embryo. The CNS, which consists of the brain and spinal cord, develops from the ectoderm. The differentiation of the ectoderm into the CNS is referred to as neurulation.

The ectoderm thickens to form the neural plate. The plate then begins to fold inwards and forms a longitudinal groove called the neural groove. The raised edges of the neural plate are called neural folds. Continuing development of the neural folds results in the folds meeting to form a tube called the neural tube (Figure 3.3). The neural tube then detaches from the surface ectoderm to lie beneath it. The tube undergoes elongation and changes in its shape. The anterior end of the neural tube develops into the brain and the posterior section becomes the spinal cord. The cavity of the neural tube becomes the central canal of the spinal cord and expands at the head to become the ventricles of the brain.

Neural tube defects

Failure of the neural tube to close correctly, leads to a group of conditions called neural tube defects (NTDs). These defects include anencephaly, encephalocele, and spina bifida. In anencephaly, the soft bony component of the skull and part of the brain are missing. Infants with anencephaly are usually stillborn or die shortly after birth. Encephalocele is herniation of the brain and meninges through a defect in the skull. The size, location, and involvement of the encephalocele will assist in determining the overall effect on the infant's physical and intellectual development. Spina bifida results from incomplete closure of the neural tube with an associated malformation of the vertebral column. The spinal cord and meninges may or may not protrude.

NTDs are among the most common, severe, congenital malformations with the United Kingdom having one of the highest rates of NTDs in the world (Medical Research Council, 1991). It is quite likely that most cases of NTD occur because of a combination of unknown genetic and environmental factors, both of which must be triggered for the NTD to occur (Seller, 1987).

Folic Acid

Folic acid (folate) is a water-soluble vitamin involved in a variety of metabolic reactions. It acts as a carrier of methyl groups and will carry one-carbon units from

Figure 3.3 – Development of the neural tube

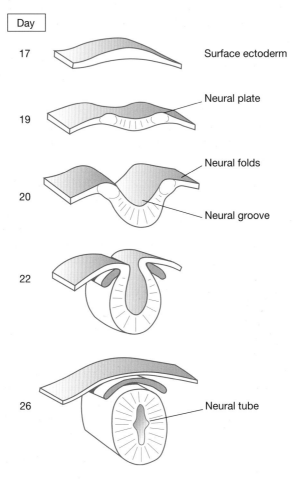

one molecule to another. The metabolism of folic acid is closely linked to that of vitamin B_{12}, and vitamin B_{12} deficiency will result in secondary folic acid deficiency (Bender, 1993). Folate deficiency affects rapidly dividing cells, particularly those of the bone marrow, intestinal mucosa, and hair follicles. Clinically, folic acid deficiency leads to a megaloblastic anaemia where large, immature red blood cells are released from the bone marrow.

Role of folic acid in prevention of NTDs

It has been suspected for some time that diet, and specifically folic acid, may have a role in the development of NTDs. Studies by Laurence *et al.* (1981) and Smithells *et al.* (1983) indicated that pre-conception folic acid or other vitamin supplementation might reduce the incidence of a recurrence of NTD in women who already have had one child with NTD. Results of work by the Medical Research

Council (1991) confirmed a link between folic acid and the development of NTDs. Providing pre-conception folic acid supplementation to women who had previously given birth to an affected infant, reduced the risk of a further such affected pregnancy by 72%.

Evidence for the role of folic acid in preventing occurrences of NTD in women expecting their first child was not clear. However, Czeizel and Dudas (1992) performed a randomised, controlled trial which concluded that a pre-conceptional multivitamin supplementation (containing folic acid) decreased the incidence of a first occurrence of NTD. In 1992, an Expert Advisory Group from the DoH published recommendations regarding folic acid supplementation and dietary folic acid, for all women planning a pregnancy.

The requirement for extra folate in relation to NTDs may be because of an interaction between a folic acid dependency and a dietary deficiency (Czeizel, 1995). Localised folic acid deficiency in the embryo may lead to impaired cell division at the time of neural tube closure. However, the actual mechanism by which folic acid assists in prevention of, but does not eliminate the risk of, NTDs still remains to be elucidated (Sadler, 1995).

Recommended requirements for folic acid during pregnancy

The reference nutrient intake (RNI) for folic acid in non-pregnant women is currently 200 μg per day.

All women who are planning a pregnancy should take a daily supplement of 400 μg folic acid from around the time of conception and for the first 3 months of pregnancy. In addition, they should try to eat 300 μg of folic acid daily. Examples of good dietary sources of folic acid can be seen in Table 3.2. Care should be taken not to overcook vegetables as this reduces their folic acid content.

Women who have unplanned pregnancies should be told to take 400 μg as soon as they realise they are pregnant, and until the twelfth week of pregnancy. Dietary intake of folic acid should also be increased to 300 μg.

Women who have had a previous pregnancy resulting in an infant with a NTD, will require a higher dose of folic acid (5 mg) and this should be taken daily until the 12th week of pregnancy. These women should also try to consume a diet with adequate folic acid.

Nursing Points

- Women with epilepsy, diabetes mellitus or other significant conditions should be encouraged to see their doctor for pre-pregnancy planning and advice.
- All women who smoke, should be strongly encouraged to stop smoking before becoming pregnant.
- The nurse may prescribe a maximum daily dose of 5 mg of folic acid.

Table 3.2 – Dietary sources of folate

Food source	µg folic acid per average serving
Bran Flakes	113
Cornflakes	88
Rice Krispies	88
All Bran	86
Brussel sprouts	127
Spinach	117
Broccoli	61
Green beans	59
Cauliflower	51
Potatoes	45
Orange juice	40
Bread (white, 2 slices)	70
Bread (granary, 2 slices)	68
Bread (wholemeal 2 slices)	29
Black-eye beans	220
Soya beans	59
Chick peas	59
Red kidney beans	44
Cottage cheese	40
Yoghurt (low fat, fruit)	24
Milk (semi-skimmed, pint)	35
Marmite	50
Bovril	50

Smoking Cessation and Nicotine Replacement Therapy (NRT)

Tobacco smoke contains over 300 chemical compounds including tars and irritants, nicotine, and carbon monoxide. These substances are responsible for the harmful effects associated with smoking. Smoking tobacco produces both short and long-term adverse effects. The short-term effects include:

- Reduced activity of cilia lining the bronchi, which decreases the removal of secretions from the lung
- An increase in carboxyhaemoglobin, which reduces the oxygen carrying capacity of the blood
- Decreased appetite
- Emotional dependence to nicotine

Long-term effects include an increased risk of

- coronary heart disease
- peripheral vascular disease

- cerebrovascular disease
- chronic obstructive pulmonary disease
- lung cancer
- peptic ulceration
- a low birth weight child at the end of pregnancy

(Waller and Renwick, 1994)

In order to reduce the burden of ill health and death that results from tobacco dependence, smoking cessation guidelines have been established for health care professionals (West *et al.*, 2000). This report concludes, along with the earlier set of guidelines (Raw *et al.*, 1998), that smoking cessation interventions delivered through the National Health Service (NHS) are an extremely cost effective way of preserving life and reducing ill health.

Two types of pharmacotherapy are available to aid smoking cessation. These are nicotine replacement therapy (NRT) and amfebutamone (bupropion). Oral amfebutamone tablets have recently been introduced as adjunctive treatment for smoking cessation, but are not available to the nurse prescriber.

Preparations for smoking cessation:

There are now six different types of NRT products available.

- Nicotine inhalator (Nicorette® inhalator)
- Nicotine lozenge (Nicotinell® lozenge)
- Nicotine medicated chewing gum (Boots® nicotine gum, Nicorette® chewing gum, Nicotinell® chewing gum)
- Nicotine nasal spray (Nicorette® nasal spray)
- Nicotine sublingual tablets (Nicorette® Microtab)
- Nicotine transdermal patches (Nicorette® patches, Boots® NRT patch, NiQuitin CQ® patches, Nicotinell® TTS patches)

Patches release nicotine over 16 or 24 h depending on manufacturer, and are available in several different doses, again depending on the manufacturer.

Mode of action

Nicotine is an agonist, and acts on nicotinic receptors in the CNS to cause neuronal excitement. Nicotine causes tolerance, physical dependence, and psychological dependence (craving) and is highly addictive (Rang *et al.*, 1995). Craving and withdrawal symptoms from nicotine include: the need to smoke, depression, irritability, insomnia, difficulty concentrating, restlessness, increased appetite, and weight gain. The peripheral effects of nicotine are due to autonomic ganglionic stimulation and include tachycardia, raised blood pressure, and reduced gut motility.

NRT products replace some of the nicotine that is normally provided by tobacco, and hence help to reduce the severity of nicotine craving and withdrawal symptoms. Nicotine is fairly short-acting and not well absorbed from the gastrointestinal tract, hence the available products largely avoid the use of the gastrointestinal tract.

Contraindications

These include: severe cardiovascular disease, recent myocardial infarction, severe cardiac arrhythmias, recent cerebrovascular accident and transient ischaemic attacks, pregnancy and breast feeding. Nicotine patches should not be used on patients with skin disease, or for use with occasional smokers.

Caution should be taken in patients with cardiovascular disease, peripheral vascular disease, diabetes mellitus, hyperthyroidism, history of gastritis/peptic ulceration and phaeochromocytoma.

Adverse effects

General adverse effects for all methods of NRT include: headache, nausea, dizziness, palpitations, dyspepsia, hiccups, insomnia, myalgia, anxiety, irritability, and poor concentration.

Adverse effects related to specific methods of administration include: skin reactions (with patches, nasal irritation and watering eyes (with nasal spray), aphthous ulceration (with inhalator and sublingual tablet), throat irritation (with spray, inhalator and sublingual tablets), cough, pharyngitis, stomatitis, sinusitis, dry mouth (with inhalator), unpleasant taste (with sublingual tablets).

Nursing Points

Important points for the nurse prescriber, reported by West *et al.* (2000) are as follows:

- There appears to be little overall difference in the effectiveness of different NRT products on smoking cessation.
- 4 mg nicotine gum may be more effective than 2 mg gum, in aiding heavy smokers (>20 cigarettes per day) to stop.
- The standard dose (21 mg) patches are more effective than the lower dose patches in medium to heavy smokers.
- There is no scientific basis for disallowing different forms of NRT to be combined, and there may be some benefit to combinations.
- There is currently insufficient research on the use of NRT in light smokers (<10 cigarettes per day), smokers under 18 years and pregnant smokers.
- NRT can be recommended for patients with cardiovascular disease, but only with agreement of the patient's physician if the disease is acute or poorly controlled.

- There is currently little scientific evidence for trying to match particular individuals to a particular NRT product. The patch however, is the most popular product with smokers.

Patients require information about dose, frequency, administration procedures, and potential adverse effects. Treatment with NRT should normally be continued for 10–12 weeks with gradual withdrawal over this period. If smoking cessation has not occurred after 3 months, treatment should be reviewed.

References

Bender DA (1993). *Introduction to Nutrition and Metabolism*. London: UCL Press.

Czeizel AE (1995). Folic acid in the prevention of neural tube defects. *Journal of Pediatric Gastroenterology and Nutrition* 20:4–16.

Czeizel AE, Dudas I (1992). Prevention of the first occurrence of neural tube defects by periconceptional vitamin supplementation. *New England Journal of Medicine* 327(26): 1832–1835.

Department of Health Expert Advisory Group (1992). *Folic acid and the prevention of neural tube defects*. London: DoH.

Galbraith A, Bullock S, Manias E, Richards A, Hunt B (1999). *Fundamentals of Pharmacology: A Text for Nurses and Health Professionals*. Singapore: Addison Wesley Longman.

Govoni LE, Hayes JE (1990). *Drugs and Nursing Implications*. New York: Prentice Hall.

Laurence KM, James N, Miller MH, Tennant GB, Cambell H (1981). Double-blind randomised controlled trial of folate treatment before conception to prevent recurrence of neural tube defects. *British Medical Journal* 282: 1509–1511.

Martini FH (2001). *Fundamentals of Anatomy and Physiology* (5th edn). Upper Saddle River: Prentice Hall.

McCance KL, Heuther SE (1994). *Pathophysiology: The Biological Basis for Disease in Adults and Children* (2nd edn). St. Louis: Mosby.

Medical Research Council Vitamin Study Research Group (1991). Prevention of neural tube defects: Results of the Medical Research Council Vitamin Study. *The Lancet* 338: 131–137.

Nathan A (1995). Analgesics. *The Pharmaceutical Journal* 255: 548–551.

Rang HP, Dale MM, Ritter JM (1995). *Pharmacology*. 3rd edn. Edinburgh: Churchill Livingstone.

Raw M, McNeill A, West R (1998). Smoking cessation guidelines for health professionals. A guide to effective smoking cessation interventions for the health care system. *Thorax* 53 (Suppl 5, Pt 1): S1–S38.

Rutishauser S (1994). *Physiology and Anatomy*. Edinburgh: Churchill Livingstone.

Sadler MJ (1995). Folic acid and NTDs – moving forwards. *BNF Nutrition Bulletin* 20: 93–95.

Seller MJ (1987). Nutritionally induced congenital defects. *Proceedings of Nutrition Society* 46(2): 227–235.

Smithells RW, Seller MJ, Harris R, Fielding DW, Schorah CJ, Nevin NC, Sheppard S, Read AP, Walker S, Wild J (1983). Further experience of vitamin supplementation for prevention of neural tube defect recurrences. *The Lancet* 1: 1027–1031.

Trounce J (1994). *Clinical Pharmacology for Nurses* (14th edn) Edinburgh: Churchill Livingstone.

Twycross R (1997). *Symptom Management in Advanced Cancer* (2nd edn). Abingdon: Radcliffe Medical Press.

Twycross R (1999). *Introducing Palliative Care* (3rd edn). Abingdon: Radcliffe Medical Press.

Waller D, Renwick A (1994). *Principles of Medical Pharmacology*. London: Balliere Tindall.

West R, McNeill A, Raw M (2000). Smoking cessation guidelines for health professionals: an update. *Thorax* 55: 987–999.

WHO (1998). *Symptom relief in terminal illness*. Geneva: WHO.

Chapter 4

Preparations for Problems and Minor Ailments of the Digestive System

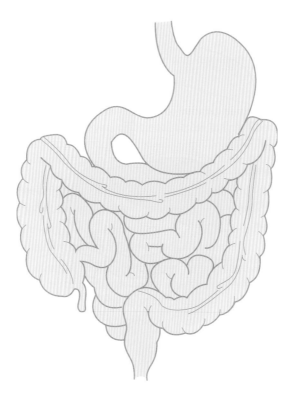

This chapter will provide the nurse prescriber with the relevant anatomy and physiology that aids understanding of the problems and ailments affecting the digestive system, together with the recommended management and treatment.

The Mouth

The mouth, also known as the oral cavity or buccal cavity, has several functions. These include:

- ingestion of food
- taste
- lubrication

Figure 4.2 – *C. albicans*: hyphae giving rise to budding yeast-like cells

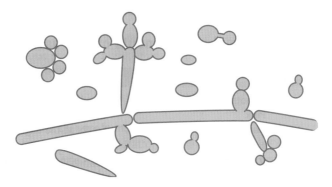

are mainly the mucosae where *C. albicans* is normally present in health, and on regions of moist skin. The infection is more commonly referred to as 'thrush'.

Patients most susceptible to opportunistic *C. albicans* include:

- pregnant women
- debilitated infants
- elderly people
- those with immunodeficiency (e.g. patients with AIDS, patients receiving cancer chemotherapy)
- those having received antibiotic or corticosteroid therapy
- those with indwelling urinary or intravenous catheters
- those with diabetes mellitus

(Brooks *et al.*, 1991)

The most common sites for *C. albicans* infection are the vagina and the mouth. Preparations listed in the NPEF allow the nurse prescriber to treat oral *Candida* and *Candida* infection of the skin and genital region (*see* Chapter 6). The oral condition is usually diagnosed following the observation of creamy white patches covering raw areas of mucous membrane and tongue within the buccal cavity. An oral swab, taken for culture and sensitivity, will provide laboratory confirmation of the infection. Diagnosis is easily made on detection of large, Gram-positive, budding yeasts (Mims *et al.*, 1993).

C. albicans particularly occurs in adults with inflammation of the corners of the mouth (angular cheilitis), ill-fitting dentures, those adults that have had prolonged antibiotic therapy and those who are immunocompromised.

In infants, the infection may be difficult to distinguish from coagulated milk lining the buccal cavity. However, diagnosis is usually apparent when attempts to remove white patches with a spatula are unsuccessful. The source of the infection in the newborn is usually from maternal vaginal infection. The infant or child may also acquire the infection from contaminated hands, bottles, teats, nipples or other articles. The infection may cause refusal to feed and may also be accompanied by fever and gastrointestinal irritation. It commonly spreads to the groin and buttocks (McCance and Huether, 1994) and these lesions should be treated with a local antifungal drug (*see* Chapter 6).

It is important before treating the infection, to try and identify the circumstances that may have lead to the infection. If the underlying problem can be corrected, for example, by improving oral hygiene or controlling blood glucose in diabetes mellitus, then the body may well be able to deal with the infection. However, treatment will shorten this process.

Preparations for the treatment of oral candidiasis:

- Fluconazole capsules and oral solution (Diflucan® capsules and oral suspension)
- Miconazole oral gel and dental lacquer (Daktarin® oral gel, Dumicoat® dental lacquer)
- Nystatin pastilles and oral suspension (Nystan® pastilles and oral suspension)

Mode of action

Miconazole and fluconazole belong to the imidazole group of antifungal agents. They are broad-spectrum drugs that act by inhibiting ergosterol synthesis in the fungal cell membrane. Ergosterol is a major constituent of the fungal cell membrane, and thus fungal growth is prevented by miconazole and fluconazole. Nystatin however, binds to ergosterol molecules in the fungal cell membrane, which alters membrane permeability and hence allows leakage of intracellular contents.

There is minimal absorption of nystatin after oral administration, with most of the drug being eliminated in faeces. However, fluconazole is very well absorbed after oral administration.

Contraindications

The contraindications for miconazole and fluconazole are hepatic impairment and previous hypersensitivity to the drug. They should be used with caution in pregnancy. They increase the activity of some other drugs when taken at the same time. These include anticoagulants (warfarin), antidiabetics (sulphonylureas) and antiepileptics (phenytoin). Miconazole antagonises the effects of amphotericin.

The only contraindication for the use of nystatin is a previous history of allergic reaction on exposure to the drug.

Adverse effects

Fluconazole may cause nausea, abdominal discomfort, flatulence, diarrhoea, liver function abnormalities, angioedema, and anaphylaxis.

Oral miconazole may produce mild gastrointestinal upset. Nausea, vomiting, and diarrhoea may occur if used for long periods. Allergy occurs only rarely. Nystatin is usually well tolerated by individuals of all age groups. Some individuals may get some oral irritation. Large doses may cause nausea, diarrhoea, and vomiting.

Nursing Points

Fluconazole capsules or oral suspension is prescribed to adults at a dose of 50 mg daily for 7–14 days for oropharyngeal candidiasis. Unusually difficult infection may be treated with 100 mg daily. Other mucosal candidal infections and severely immunocompromised patients may require 50 mg of fluconazole for 14–30 days.

In adults, miconazole gel 5–10 ml should be applied 6 hourly for 10 days, or for up to 2 days after the symptoms have cleared. Children over 6 years of age require 5 ml, four times daily, whilst children under 2 years are prescribed 2.5 ml twice daily. The gel is applied after food and should be retained in the mouth for as long as possible. Patients may require information about hand hygiene. Hands should be washed before and after application. Contact with the eyes and nose should be avoided when applying miconazole. Patients with Candida-associated denture stomatitis require dental lacquer containing miconazole 50 mg/g. The contents of a 1 g bottle should be applied to the upper surface of the upper denture after thorough cleansing, allowed to dry and then replaced. This should be repeated twice at intervals of 1 week.

The dose of nystatin for both adults and children is the same. The dose of oral suspension is 100,000 U (1 ml) four times daily after food, or one pastille four times daily after food. Patients with immunosuppression may need higher doses up to 500,000 U four times daily. Those taking the oral suspension should be instructed to place 0.5 ml inside each cheek, and then keep in the mouth for as long as possible before swallowing. Nystatin should be continued for 2 days after the infection has resolved. As for miconazole, good hand hygiene is important.

Patients with dental prostheses, that have oral *C. albicans* infection, should soak them in chlorhexidene for 10 min in order to reduce the risk of reinfecting the mouth with contaminated dentures (Mallet and Bailey, 1996).

Measures to control *C. albicans* in infants and children include: rinsing the infant's mouth with plain water after each feed and before applying medication, sterilisation of feeding bottles, teats and pacifiers. Infants with candidal nappy dermatitis can introduce yeast into the mouth from contaminated hands. The placing of clothing over the nappy can prevent the cycle of re-infection.

Patients should be encouraged to take the preparation for the prescribed period.

The nurse may prescribe thymol glycerin for patients that require a general mouthwash to freshen the mouth, or to assist in the relief of pain from traumatic ulceration. The mouthwash is diluted with warm water and used as required for general oral hygiene. It may be used at frequent intervals until the discomfort and inflammation of ulceration subsides.

Stomatitis

Stomatitis is inflammation of the mucosa of the mouth. Both gingivitis and glossitis are forms of stomatitis. Stomatitis may be caused by one of the many diseases of the mouth or it may accompany another disease. A common cause of stomatitis is candidiasis and the reader should consult the earlier material in this chapter for its treatment.

The Salivary Glands

There are three pairs of salivary glands which secrete saliva into the oral cavity. The parotid salivary glands produce a thick secretion containing large amounts of salivary amylase. The sublingual salivary glands produce a watery, mucous secretion that acts as a buffer and lubricant. The submandibular salivary glands secrete a mixture of buffers, mucins, and salivary amylase.

Each day, these glands collectively produce 1.0–1.5 l of saliva. The majority of saliva is water (approximately 99%) with the remainder comprising electrolytes, buffers, glycoproteins (mucins), antibodies, enzymes, and waste material. There is a continuous low level secretion of saliva which washes over the oral surfaces keeping them clean. The pH of saliva is 6.8–7.0 due to buffers and this prevents a buildup of acids caused by bacterial activity. IgA antibodies and lysozymes also help control the numbers of oral bacteria.

Should the quantity of salivary secretions fall, due to factors such as emotional distress, radiation exposure, and limited or no oral food/drink intake, then bacterial proliferation is likely. Recurring infections and progressive erosion of the teeth and gums is then a likely outcome (Martini, 2001).

Ingestion of food produces saliva with several functions: lubrication of the mouth, lubrication and moistening of materials in the mouth, dissolution of chemicals that can stimulate taste buds and finally initiation of the digestion of carbohydrates via the action of salivary amylase. In addition to food, any object in the mouth can stimulate a salivary reflex. Also the smell of food, thinking about food and chewing with an empty mouth will all initiate an increase in salivary secretion rates.

Dry mouth

Xerostomia or dryness of the mouth is a common problem observed in patients and can result from:

- Sjögren's syndrome
- medication (antiparkinsonian, antihistamines, lithium, monoamine oxidase inhibitors, tricyclic antidepressants, and clonidine)
- radiotherapy
- psychogenic causes
- dehydration, shock, and renal failure

(Kumar and Clark, 1998)

Following oral assessment, dehydration, oral candidiasis, and aphthous ulceration should be treated (see relevant earlier sections in this chapter). Medication responsible for xerostomia should be discontinued if possible. General measures to be undertaken include regular oral care, sucking ice or pineapple chunks, and using artificial saliva. A balanced artificial saliva should be of neutral pH and contain electrolytes corresponding to the composition of saliva. Several proprietary preparations are available including Luborant®, Salivace®, Saliveze®, and others.

The Oesophagus and Stomach

The oesophagus is a hollow muscular tube approximately 25 cm long and 2 cm in diameter at its widest point. Its main function is to transport food and liquids into the stomach. The oesophagus begins at the level of the cricoid cartilage and is inferior to the larynx and dorsal to the trachea. It passes through the mediastinum penetrating the diaphragm at an opening called the oesophageal hiatus. After 3–4 cm it meets the stomach at an opening called the cardiac orifice. Resting muscle tone in the circular muscle in the superior 3 cm of the oesophagus normally prevents air from entering the oesophagus. The inferior end of the oesophagus normally remains in a state of active contraction. This prevents backflow of materials from the stomach into the oesophagus. Neither region has a well-defined sphincter muscle compared to those that can be identified in other parts of the digestive tract. However, the terms upper oesophageal sphincter and lower oesophageal sphincter (cardiac sphincter) are often used to describe these regions of the oesophagus (Martini, 2001).

Below the oesophagus, the gastrointestinal tract expands to form the temporary storage tank called the stomach. The inner surface of the stomach is thrown into a series of folds called rugae, which increase the surface area of the mucosa. The mucosal surface consists of a layer of mucus-secreting epithelial cells, but this is interrupted by multiple openings, each of which leads down to a tubular gastric gland or 'gastric pit' (see Figure 4.3). The upper one-third of each pit consists of many mucus-secreting neck cells. Mucus forms an acid-resistant layer over the mucosa. Deeper down in the pit are found parietal cells, which secrete hydrochloric acid (causing a stomach pH of 2–3), and chief cells which secrete the enzyme precursor pepsinogen. The gastric mucosa also contains G cells which produce the hormone gastrin and histaminocytes secreting the chemical histamine.

Heartburn

Heartburn is a retrosternal or epigastric burning sensation that spreads upwards to the throat. The pain can spread to the neck, across the chest and may be misinterpreted as pain resulting from cardiac ischaemia. It may occur at night, or when an individual has bent or stooped. The pain may be precipitated by alcohol and hot drinks. Heartburn is a common symptom of acid reflux and is often trivial (Kumar and Clark, 1998).

Non-drug measures should be recommended to patients as these may be of use in mild cases. These should include:

- weight loss in overweight/obese patients
- cessation of smoking

Figure 4.3 – Structure of a gastric gland

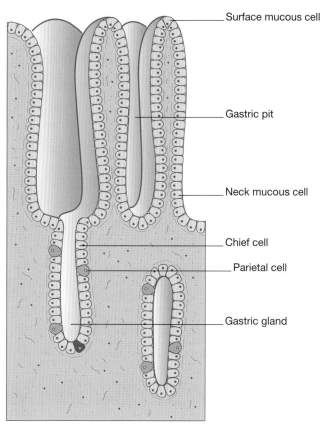

- Surface mucous cell
- Gastric pit
- Neck mucous cell
- Chief cell
- Parietal cell
- Gastric gland

- reduction in alcohol consumption
- raising the head of the bed at night
- avoidance of meals late at night
- avoiding foods which the patient finds worsens the symptoms
- avoiding large meals

Mild to moderate heartburn will often respond to antacids and alginate-antacids. Many people with symptoms of reflux, control them with antacids and alginates purchased over-the-counter. Antacids are bases that raise the gastric luminal pH by neutralising hydrochloric acid. Alginate-antacids, which are derived from seaweed, form a floating raft on top of the gastric contents and therefore present a barrier to reflux and protect the oesophageal mucosa.

For individuals with mild to moderate heartburn that have no or a minimal response to antacids and alginates, the nurse prescriber may prescribe the use of an H_2-receptor antagonist. Patients with persistent or recurrent heartburn and those who meet the referral criteria for suspected cancer (DoH, 2000) should be referred to a physician.

Urgent referral guidelines for upper gastrointestinal cancers are summarised as follows:

- Food sticking on swallowing at any age
- Dyspepsia at any age together with one or more of the following:
  - weight loss
  - anaemia
  - vomiting
- Dyspepsia in patients aged 55 years or more with at least one of the following:
  - onset of dyspepsia less than a year ago
  - continuous symptoms since onset
- Dyspepsia combined with at least one of the following:
  - family history of an upper gastrointestinal cancer in more than two first degree relatives
  - Barrett's oesophagus
  - pernicious anaemia
  - peptic ulcer surgery over 20 years ago
  - known dysplasia, atrophic gastritis, intestinal metaplasia
- Jaundice
- Upper abdominal mass

(DoH, 2000)

Preparations for the treatment of heartburn:

The NPEF has included the following H_2-receptor antagonist drugs for patients with mild to moderate heartburn:

- Cimetidine tablets, effervescent tablets, suspension, and syrup (Cimetidine tablets; Dyspamet® suspension; Tagamet® tablets, effervescent tablets and syrup)
- Famotidine tablets (Pepcid® tablets)
- Nizatidine capsules (Nizatidine capsules, Axid® capsules)
- Ranitidine tablets, effervescent tablets and syrup (Ranitidine tablets; Zantac® tablets, effervescent tablets, and syrup)

Mode of action

Although gastric acid production is generally not increased, drug therapy relies heavily upon suppression of gastric acid secretion in order to reduce the volume and raise the pH of stomach contents refluxing into the oesophagus (Drugs and Therapeutic Bulletin, 1996). Binding of histamine, gastrin, and acetylcholine to parietal cell membrane receptors leads to hydrochloric acid secretion into the stomach lumen. H_2-receptor antagonists bind to and block the histamine receptor sites of the parietal cells resulting in reduced acid secretion.

Contraindications

This group of drugs should be used with caution in hepatic impairment, renal impairment, pregnancy, and breast feeding.

Cimetidine has drug metabolism inhibitory properties and should be avoided in patients stabilised on warfarin, phenytoin, aminophylline, and theophylline. Famotidine, nizatidine, and ranitidine do not however, share these properties.

Adverse effects

These include diarrhoea and other gastrointestinal disturbances, altered liver function tests, headache, rash, dizziness, and tiredness.

Rare adverse effects may include bradycardia, atrio-ventricular block, acute pancreatitis, confusion, depression, hallucinations in the elderly, hypersensitivity reactions, blood disorders, gynaecomastia, and impotence.

Nursing Points

A full assessment of the patient's history of symptoms, dietary intake, eating patterns, use of alcohol, caffeine, and tobacco, and attempts at life-style changes and self-medication should be made.

The nurse prescriber should give advice on life-style modifications and the use of antacids and alginates. H_2-receptor antagonists may be prescribed as appropriate.

Patients should be informed that H_2-receptor antagonists need to be taken before meals to decrease food-induced acid secretion. Patients should also refrain from smoking and drinking alcohol as these activities impede the effectiveness of the drug.

Reduced doses may be required by elderly patients as they have reduced gastric acid.

Failure to resolve symptoms with antacids, alginates and H_2-receptor antagonists usually then requires proton pump inhibitor drugs. These are not available to the independent nurse prescriber, and patients should at this point be referred to a physician.

Nausea and vomiting in palliative care

Independent nurse prescribers working in palliative care are able to prescribe a number of products that may relieve nausea and vomiting associated with cancer and chemotherapy treatment. Treatment will depend on the cause, with 80% of cases being due to gastric stasis, intestinal obstruction, drugs, and biochemical factors. Raised intracranial pressure accounts for less than 5% of cases of nausea and vomiting (Twycross, 2000).

Figure 4.4 – Section through the small intestine

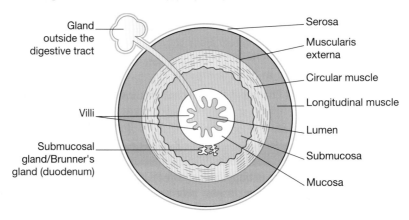

The wall of the small intestine has the same general structure as other organs of the digestive system. However, there are regional specialisations (see Figure 4.4).

The lining of the small intestine has many transverse folds called plicae. In addition, the mucosa of the small intestine has many finger-like projections called villi. Each villus is covered by epithelial cells whose exposed surfaces contain microvilli, also referred to as a 'brush border'. This arrangement increases the total area for absorption by a factor of more than 600, to approximately 2 million/cm^2 (Martini, 2001).

The main functions of the small intestine are the enzymatic degradation of nutrient molecules into simpler component molecules, and the absorption of these digestion products, along with water, minerals, and vitamins, from the gut lumen into the blood. In order for these processes to occur, the small intestine secretes approximately 1.8 l of intestinal juice into the gut lumen, in addition to the digestive secretions (bile and pancreatic juice) from the liver and pancreas respectively.

Three types of motility are seen in the small intestine which aid digestion and absorption. Segmentation involves no travelling wave of contraction. This allows for mixing of contents and promotes efficient digestion and absorption. Peristalsis provides the main propulsive force, but the waves of contraction only travel a short distance before dying out. This means that small intestinal contents travel slowly, therefore aiding digestion and absorption. Propulsive migratory motor complexes develop in the fasted state when absorption is complete. These assist the movement of the intestinal residue from the ileum into the large intestine via the ileocaecal valve.

Failure to absorb any component of ingested food is referred to as malabsorption. This may arise from defects of digestion as well as faults with the absorption process itself.

Gastroenteritis

Gastroenteritis is caused by infection in the gastro-intestinal tract which usually results in abdominal pain and diarrhoea of acute onset and short duration, and commonly occurs with vomiting (Travis *et al.*, 1998). Additional symptoms may include abdominal cramps, bloating, flatulence, nausea, fever, faecal urgency, and tenesmus. Those most susceptible include the very young, the elderly, patients with immunodeficiency and patients with conditions causing gastric hypochlorhydria. Some patients may report that they have recently travelled abroad, eaten at a mass catering event, eaten take-away food, consumed poultry or seafood or had food they felt was undercooked. These factors are all common causes of food poisoning.

Uncomplicated acute gastroenteritis does not usually need investigation, because it usually resolves rapidly and spontaneously within a few days (Travis *et al.*, 1998; Griffin *et al.*, 1999). Assessment of hydration, fluid replacement, antimotility agents and patient education should be provided to patients with uncomplicated acute gastroenteritis. Common symptoms of mild dehydration produced by gastroenteritis result from combined water and salt loss, and include lassitude, anorexia, nausea, light headedness, and postural hypotension (Farthing *et al.*, 1996). Advice and encouragement about rehydrating should be given. The young and frail elderly are particularly susceptible to becoming dehydrated and the use of oral rehydration solution (ORS) is advisable (Avery and Snyder, 1990; Bennett and Greenough, 1987; Murphy, 1998). Proprietary solutions include Dioralyte®, Electrolade®, and Rehidrat® and these should be used to rehydrate over 3–4 h. Once rehydration has occurred, further dehydration should be prevented by encouraging the patient to drink normal volumes of fluid, and by replacing continuing losses with an ORS. Infants should be offered breast milk or a formula feed in between ORS drinks.

Preparations for the management of gastroenteritis:

Antimotility agents are used to some effect in providing symptomatic relief from diarrhoea as a result of gastroenteritis. Those available to the nurse prescriber are

- Codeine phosphate tablets (*see* page 30 – Schedule drugs)
- Loperamide capsules and syrup

Mode of action

These are narcotic analgesics, which act upon opioid μ-receptors on myenteric neurones in the gut wall. Acetylcholine release is inhibited from these neurones and this in turn decreases peristaltic movements and hence, decreases bowel motility. Forward movements of bowel contents are slowed allowing for some reabsorption, thus increasing the viscosity of the bowel contents and correcting the diarrhoea (Galbraith *et al.*, 1999). These drugs are useful in non-infectious diarrhoea. However, in infective gastroenteritis, the diarrhoea is a protective mechanism that is trying to rid the body of the invading pathogen. Use of antimotility drugs in this situation is not recommended. In addition, the use of antimotility drugs in infants and children with gastroenteritis should be avoided. They have not been shown to be useful and have also been associated with serious adverse effects including central nervous system toxicity and ileus (Murphy, 1998; AAP, 1996).

Contraindications

Codeine phosphate should not be used if patients have: hypersensitivity to opioids, respiratory depression, severe respiratory disease, acute alcoholism and where there is risk of paralytic ileus.

Loperamide should not be administered to patients where inhibition of peristalsis should be avoided, where abdominal distention develops or in conditions such as active ulcerative colitis.

Adverse effects

Codeine phosphate may cause: drowsiness, sedation, dizziness, agitation, dependency, lethargy, hallucinations, mood changes, bradycardia, palpitations, hypotension, tachycardia, dry mouth, miosis, nausea, anorexia, constipation, urinary retention, flushing, rash, urticaria, sweating, pruritus, hypothermia, and respiratory depression.

Loperamide is a synthetic opioid which cannot readily cross the blood-brain barrier. Main adverse effects include: abdominal cramps, dizziness, drowsiness, skin reactions, paralytic ileus, and abdominal bloating.

Nursing Points

Obtain a full history from the patient to assess what may have been responsible for the symptoms of their gastroenteritis. Also assess their state of hydration, and frequency and consistency of bowel motions.

Further investigations may be required if the patient is elderly, more than one person is affected, symptoms have persisted for more than 4 days and there are additional sequelae (Travis et al., 1998). Patients presenting with fever, bloody diarrhoea, abdominal pain and tenesmus, severe dehydration, faecal incontinence, vomiting such that they are unable to retain an ORS, shock and protracted diarrhoea must be referred to a physician for assessment (Farthing et al., 1996).

Teach the patient to keep the peri-anal region clean to avoid skin irritation.

Meticulous hand hygiene and use of a personal towel should be emphasised.

All cases of gastroenteritis should be regarded as infectious. A liquid stool is likely to cause contamination of the hands and the environment, causing the spread of the faecal organisms. All cases should be kept away from work or school until the patient is free of diarrhoea and vomiting (Farthing et al., 1996).

Antibiotics are only useful in certain specific infections. These include infections by *Salmonella, Shigella, Campylobacter*, and *Clostridia* species where diarrhoea may be very severe. In most cases a positive stool culture should be obtained and antibiotic sensitivity tests performed. Nurse prescribers are not able to prescribe antibiotics to treat gastroenteritis.

Bowel colic in palliative care

Nurse prescribers in palliative care are able to treat bowel colic in patients with cancer. Bowel colic refers to an attack of abdominal pain caused by spasmodic contractions of the intestine.

Preparation for the management of bowel colic:

- Hyoscine butylbromide injection (Buscopan®)

Mode of action
This is an antimuscarinic (anticholinergic) drug with smooth muscle relaxant properties and which will also reduce gastrointestinal secretions.

Contraindications

Hyoscine butylbromide should be avoided in patients with hypersensitivity, prostatic hypertrophy, pyloric stenosis, paralytic ileus, urinary retention, closed-angle glaucoma, and porphyria.

Adverse effects

These include depression, confusion, blurred vision, photophobia, dilated pupils, raised ocular pressure, palpitations, bradycardia, tachycardia, arrythmias, flushing, dryness of the skin, dry mouth, constipation, difficulty swallowing, and urinary retention.

Nursing Points

Check the patient's medical history based on the list of contraindications.

Regularly monitor bowel sounds, an absence indicating decreased motility and risk of paralytic ileus. Monitor also for constipation due to decreased gut motility.

Boiled sweets, ice chips or chewing gum may help to deal with the dry mouth which may result from treatment.

Thread Worms

Anthelmintics are drugs used to eradicate helminthiasis or infestation by helminths (parasitic worms). In the United Kingdom, the nurse prescriber may need to prescribe treatment for either thread worms, or in rare instances, roundworms, both of which are found within the digestive tract.

Both of these infestations constitute parasitic diseases and the human host derives no benefit from their presence. This is unlike the symbiotic relationship seen, for example, between man and colonic flora. Removal of the parasites is essential to prevent a continuous cycle of infection in the patient and to prevent spread to other individuals.

Helminths are multicellular parasitic worms that can be classified as nematodes (roundworms), cestodes (tapeworms), and trematodes (flatworms or flukes). Helminths may infect humans by ingestion, skin penetration or injection by insects. Their life cycles vary from simple to complex and are useful in understanding the pathophysiology and treatment of infection. The signs and symptoms of helminthiasis are specific for each helminth but reflect disturbances to specific organs or systems. Disturbances may include invasion and destruction of tissue, toxin production, obstruction, competition with the host for nutrients and hypersensitivity reactions.

Helminth infections in patients that can be treated by the nurse are due to the nematodes *Enterobius vermicularis*, known as the thread worm or pinworm and, more rarely, *Ascaris lumbricoides*, which is commonly called the roundworm. These nematodes are cylindrical and elongated with tapered ends.

In the UK, it has been estimated that about 40% of children under 10 years of age suffer from a thread worm infestation. Schoolchildren are most commonly affected, probably due to more frequent hand-to-mouth contact (Li Wan Po and Li Wan Po, 1992). Transmission rates are particularly high in dense populations living under conditions of poor sanitation.

Thread worms are the only commonly seen helminths in the UK. The roundworm has a much lower incidence and is more likely to have been contracted abroad. There are potentially serious consequences arising from roundworm infection, and patients should be referred to their General Practitioner if it is suspected (Nathan, 1997). Complications of a heavy roundworm infestation may include intestinal obstruction and pulmonary eosinophilia.

Due to the higher incidence of thread worms in the UK, this section will concentrate on their treatment and management.

Life cycle

The life cycle of the thread worm is shown in Figure 4.5. Infection occurs usually from contact with ova present in food or water or on bedlinen and clothing. The ova are ingested and the worms develop in the small intestine. The adult worms then migrate into the colon. Gravid female worms move through the large bowel and then lay their eggs in the peri-anal region. The subsequent intense itching that occurs means that ova are collected under the finger nails as a result of scratching. The ova may then be returned to the mouth directly or indirectly in food. This autoinfection maintains the parasite in the host. Others may be infected by consuming food or contacting bed clothing, bed linen or towels to which eggs have adhered. The adult worms only survive for up to 6 weeks and for the development of new worms, ova must be swallowed and exposed to the action of

Figure 4.5 – Life cycle of the thread worm

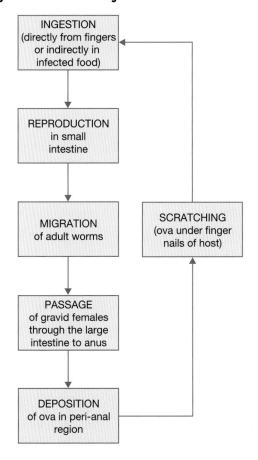

digestive secretions of the upper intestinal tract via the mechanisms described above.

Clinical features

Severe pruritus ani is the usual symptom that thread worms are present. Itching is particularly common at night-time and disrupts sleep. When symptoms are present, the worms, which are 8–12 mm long, may be visible on the peri-anal skin or on the stools. There may be considerable discomfort and irritability in young children. Females may also present with vulvo-vaginitis and a vaginal discharge.

Diagnosis is based on the presence of these symptoms together with identification of a female worm or ova in the peri-anal region or on faeces. A swab should be obtained without washing the skin beforehand or alternatively a small piece of adhesive tape may be applied to the peri-anal skin. Either of these procedures should be undertaken in the morning on rising.

Preparations for the treatment of thread worms:

- Mebendazole tablets (Ovex®, Vermox®)
- Mebendazole oral suspension (Vermox® oral suspension)
- Piperazine citrate elixir
- Piperazine and senna powder (Pripsen® oral powder)

Mode of action

Mebendazole is considered a broad-spectrum anthelmintic. This is the drug of choice for adults and children over 2 years of age. The drug has its effect by interfering with the microtubule system of the worm. Glucose uptake into the worm is prevented and therefore glucose distribution throughout the worm is affected. Eventually the worm's energy stores become depleted and the worm becomes immobilised or dies. It will then be expelled from the gastrointestinal tract after several days. Mebendazole acts locally within the gastrointestinal tract and less than 10% of the drug is systemically absorbed. The remainder is excreted unchanged in faeces.

Piperazine, also available to nurse prescribers, tends to be the drug of second choice, when mebendazole is not a suitable option for some patients. Piperazine causes paralysis of the worm by blocking the action of the neurotransmitter acetylcholine, at the neuromuscular junction. It may enhance the activity of a second neurotransmitter, gamma-aminobutyric acid (GABA), which also leads to paralysis. Normal peristaltic activity in the intestine then aids removal of the worm.

Pripsen® oral powder contains the stimulant laxative, senna, to enhance expulsion of the worm. Piperazine is described as a vermifuge, as the worms are paralysed, then expelled alive. A vermicide however, will kill the worm, as in the case of mebendazole.

Contraindications

Mebendazole should not be used in pregnancy as it crosses the placenta and teratogenesis, or deformity in embryos, has been demonstrated in rats. It should not be prescribed for children under 2 years, as there is inadequate information available about its use in this age group.

Piperazine may be taken in pregnancy, but preferably under the supervision of a physician. It should be avoided in the first trimester, and in addition, lactating women should not breast feed their infant within 8 h of taking a dose of piperazine. The drug should be avoided in patients with renal disease, liver disease and epilepsy. As piperazine lowers a patient's seizure threshold, it should not be used with other drugs that also do this, for example, the phenothiazines.

Adverse effects

Mebendazole is considered to be virtually free of adverse effects with rare occurrences of diarrhoea and abdominal pain.

Adverse effects of piperazine include nausea, vomiting, diarrhoea, anorexia, abdominal cramps, blurred vision, rash, bronchospasm, and more rarely, drowsiness, muscular incoordination, and convulsions.

Nursing Points

In adults and children over 2 years, mebendazole is given as a single 100 mg dose.

Re-infection is common and a second dose may be given after 2–3 weeks. It does not need to be given with food and the tablet form of the drug may be chewed.

Piperazine can be used in children under 2 years. It is usually given daily for 7 days, followed by a second course 7 days later.

Although senna is present in Pripsen®, an additional laxative may be required if the patient is constipated.

Drug therapy is crucial if the infestation is to be successfully eradicated. However, prevention of re-infection is a major priority. Other important issues include treating the whole family at the same time as the patient. Other individuals may be infected but are still asymptomatic at that time.

All individuals possibly infected should cut their fingernails short. Hand washing and nail scrubbing is essential after using the toilet, before preparing/handling food, and before eating.

A bath or shower should be taken on rising in the morning. This aims to wash away any eggs that may have been laid during the night.

In order to prevent scratching, pants or pyjamas should be worn at night. These must be washed daily to remove and destroy eggs that may be present. Cotton mittens or gloves can be worn by children as repeated scratching is a problem. Mittens too, must be laundered daily.

The Large Intestine

The large intestine or large bowel (Figure 4.6) is approximately 1.5 m long and 7.5 cm wide in the adult and consists of three main parts: the caecum, colon, and rectum. The caecum receives approximately 500 ml of food material or chyme each day from the ileum via the ileo-caecal valve. The caecum is a blind-ending pouch from which the vermiform appendix projects. The appendix serves no specific function in humans, whilst the caecum collects and stores chyme, before it is moved on into the ascending colon. The ascending colon passes up the right side of the abdomen towards the liver, where it turns at the hepatic flexure or right colic flexure, to become the transverse colon. At the splenic or left colic flexure, the colon turns down the left side of the abdomen as the descending colon. At the iliac fossa the colon then curves at the sigmoid flexure as the sigmoid or pelvic colon. This then becomes the rectum from which the anus forms the exit from the large intestine.

Figure 4.6 – Anatomy of the large intestine

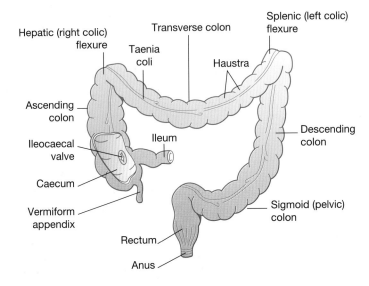

The wall of the large intestine generally has the same structure as the other organs of the digestive tract. However, the mucosa is not folded to form villi, as in the small intestine, and has a smooth absorptive surface composed mainly of columnar epithelial cells and mucus-secreting goblet cells. The muscularis externa or muscle layer does have an inner circular layer but lacks a continuous layer of longitudinal smooth muscle, unlike the rest of the tract. The muscles are organised into three flat bands called taeniae coli. Because the taeniae coli are not as long as the colon itself, the wall of the intestine becomes puckered, forming pouches called haustra.

Functions

Absorption of water and salt

Sodium is actively absorbed from the ascending and transverse colon and both chloride and water follow passively. Approximately 350 ml will be reabsorbed from the initial 500 ml of chyme entering the colon. This leaves 150 g of faecal material to be eliminated, consisting of 100 g of water and 50 g of solids (undigested cellulose, bilirubin, bacteria, and a small amount of salt). The amount of water reabsorbed from the colon will depend on the length of time the food residue remains.

Mucus secretion

An alkaline mucus solution is secreted which contains bicarbonate and maintains the colonic pH at 7.5–8.0. The bicarbonate protects the mucosa by neutralising acids produced by bacterial fermentation. The mucus lubricates the faeces to facilitate their passage through the intestine.

Movement and storage of faeces

For the majority of the time, peristaltic movements of the large intestine tend to be slow, and non-propulsive, therefore aiding absorption and storage functions.

Haustral contractions, which occur at intervals of approximately 30 min shuffle the contents back and forth along the large intestine. These contractions are largely controlled by local reflexes involving the intrinsic nerve plexuses (submucosal plexus and myenteric plexus). However, 3–4 times a day, large contractions called mass movements occur, which drive the colonic contents forward into the distal part of the large intestine, for storage in the rectum. Mass movements arise because of the gastro-colic reflex. Food entering the stomach at mealtimes causes release of the hormone gastrin, which enhances colonic motility, together with extrinsic autonomic nervous system activity.

Defaecation

Distention of the rectum as a result of mass movements stimulates stretch receptors in the rectal wall and initiates the defaecation reflex. This causes a strong urge to defaecate, sometimes referred to as the 'call to stool'. Relaxation of the smooth muscle of the internal anal sphincter and relaxation of the skeletal muscle of the external anal sphincter will permit defaecation. There is voluntary control over the skeletal muscle of the external sphincter and should the circumstances for defaecation not be satisfactory, an individual can prevent defaecation despite the defaecation reflex. The urge to defaecate will then subside following relaxation of the rectal wall.

Bacterial activity

Many species of bacteria colonize the large intestine and form a symbiotic relationship with man where each derives some benefit from the other. However, these natural bowel flora or commensals may become pathogenic if they are introduced into another part of the body. These bacteria synthesize vitamins K and B_{12} in small amounts and ferment some food residues to produce gas or flatus. Bacteria, both alive and dead, may make up as much as fifty percent of the dry weight of faeces.

Under normal circumstances, the functions of the large intestine previously described, will enable the continued production, temporary storage and successful elimination of semi-solid faeces. This contributes to the maintenance of internal homeostasis and general feelings of well-being for the individual. Disruption of these processes can cause constipation.

Constipation

Constipation refers to the difficult passage of stools. This may be due to an abnormality of stool bulk, hardness, or frequency, causing them to be difficult to expel. The reasons for constipation are multifaceted but focus on the following issues.

The volume of faecal material

If an individual's diet is rich in fibre, the volume of faecal material is great, and stools are large and bulky. These large bulky stools stimulate peristalsis in the colon, and faeces are propelled into the rectum innervating the neuromuscular responses of defaecation. Correspondingly, diets that are inadequate in fibre give rise to smaller, less bulky stools, which can predispose to constipation.

Transit time

Transit time is the time taken for stools to travel through the colon and is dependent upon the muscular activity of the colon. It can be affected by certain disorders and medications. Stools that have an increased transit time, i.e. travel slowly through the colon, allow a greater reabsorption of water. This, in turn, results in a smaller volume of faecal material, which further increases transit time. This smaller volume of faecal material can give rise to constipation.

Anatomical integrity

A mass in the lumen of the colon may completely or partially obstruct the passage of stools. In complete obstruction there will be an absence of faeces. If the lumen is partially obstructed, transit time will be increased and the characteristics of the stools may be altered. Disorders affecting anatomical integrity are curable but also life threatening. Therefore, it is essential that these disorders be detected.

Defaecation

To defaecate, the rectum must initially become filled with faeces and stimulate sensory receptors in the walls of the rectum and anal canal. Disruption of the process of defaecation at any stage can result in constipation. For example, multiple sclerosis or spinal cord injury will disrupt the sensation of a distended rectum.

Nursing assessment

To be able to accurately identify the presence and cause of constipation, an accurate assessment of the patient is essential. This assessment should cover the following areas.

History

A critical aspect of assessment is the history of the constipation. Has the patient had problems with constipation for several years, or are the changes in bowel pattern recent? Carcinoma of the colon, if detected at an early stage, is curable and may only present with altered bowel habits. Therefore, it is important that recent changes are identified. Other reasons for constipation may be a change in fluid intake, poor posture or a reduction in exercise levels. A change in routine bowel pattern and postponement of the urge to defecate will also perpetuate constipation.

Accompanying symptoms

Symptoms accompanying constipation, and when these symptoms begin, need to be identified. Increased bowel sounds, abdominal distention and pain may be a sign of a structural lesion. Pencil shaped thinner stools could indicate a lower lesion in the descending colon. An abdominal mass, weight loss, fatigue, and jaundice can each be associated with colon carcinoma of an advanced stage. Non-specific discomfort can also be seen with the intermittent obstruction of a colon cancer. Stools that are black, or malaena, suggests a higher intestinal lesion. Colonic bleeding may be indicated if blood is mixed in with the stools. If stools are covered with blood, this may point to lower colonic and rectal disease, whereas blood on the toilet paper is indicative of anal fissure or haemorrhoids.

Constipation is also a frequent companion of depression. Therefore, it is important to look for lethargy, fatigue and other symptoms that may indicate that the patient is depressed.

Family and personal medical history

An important consideration is the patient's medical history and the identification of any factors that may predispose to constipation. It is also important to ascertain whether there is a family history of colorectal carcinoma.

Medication

Certain medications, for example opiates, aluminium antacids, and anticholinergics can cause constipation. If the patient is taking any such preparations these need to be identified. Drugs, especially laxatives, are a major cause in the development of long standing constipation. Gradually, over time, frequent use of laxatives may reduce intestinal muscle tone, and the propulsive function of the colon is impaired. The end result is an atonic, non-functioning colon.

Physical examination

Weight loss, cachexia, and malnutrition could be signs of carcinoma or depression. A tender abdomen with guarding, rigidity, with rebound tenderness and absent bowel sounds, indicates an acute condition, perhaps requiring surgical consultation. If an abdominal mass is evident, this could suggest structural disease. If a rectal examination is undertaken, a full rectum suggests sensory deficit nerve damage or chronic failure to heed the urge to defecate. Absence of stool suggests a more chronic obstruction or laxative abuse.

Primary management

Constipation can often be treated successfully with non-pharmacological methods, and this should be the first step in the management of this problem. Patient education, therefore, plays a vital role in the management of constipation. An increase in the consumption of dietary fibre and daily fluid intake, where appropriate, should always be considered and implemented. The ideal quantity of fibre intake per day is 18–30 g (DoH, 1991). The patient needs to be encouraged to eat foods such as peas, beans, brussel sprouts, wholemeal bread, wholemeal pasta, bran breakfast cereals, and muesli. These foods all contain more than 4 g of fibre per portion, which will help to provide a fibre-rich diet. Following an increased fibre intake, individuals may experience bloating or flatulence, and it is important to stress that this will usually resolve in a week or so. If patients are not keen to change their eating habits, bran in an unprocessed form will also help to increase fibre intake. Unless contraindicated, due to the presence of other pathology, it is important that at least 1.5–2.0 l of fluid are taken each day and that exercise is undertaken. It is also essential that patients are encouraged to respond to the defaecation reflex. Ignoring the reflex means that further water will be reabsorbed from the colonic lumen making stools difficult to pass. Encouragement should therefore be given to use the toilet shortly after mealtimes.

Secondary management

Patients that do not respond to primary measures to alleviate their constipation, or who are already in discomfort because of it, are likely to require drug therapy in the form of a laxative or rectal preparation. Laxatives are medicines that promote a bowel action and have various synonyms to describe them. Those producing a mild effect are sometimes referred to as aperients whilst those producing a strong effect may be called a purgative or cathartic. Rectal preparations refer to medicines in the form of a suppository or enema.

Preparations for the treatment of constipation:

These are listed in Table 4.2. These products are usually classified according to their mode of action and will be described in the following section.

Table 4.2 – Laxatives and rectal preparations available to the nurse prescriber

Group of laxatives	Generic name
Bulk-forming	Isphagula husk granules
	Isphagula husk granules effervescent
	Isphagula husk powder
	Sterculia granules
	Sterculia and frangula granules
Osmotic	Lactulose solution
	Lactitol powder
	Macrogol powder
	Magnesium hydroxide mixture
	Phosphate enema
	Sodium citrate enemas
Stimulant	Senna granules
	Senna oral solution
	Senna tablets
	Senna and Isphagula granules
	Bisacodyl tablets
	Bisacodyl suppositories
	Codanthramer capsules
	Codanthramer capsules, strong
	Codanthramer oral suspension
	Codanthramer oral suspension, strong
	Codanthrusate capsules
	Codanthrusate oral suspension
	Sodium picosulfate elixir
	Glycerol suppositories
Faecal softeners	Arachis oil retention enema
	Docusate capsules
	Docusate enema
	Docusate oral solution

Bulk-forming laxatives

- Isphagula (Fybogel®, Regulan®)
- Sterculia (Normacol®, Normacol plus®)

These drugs are effective in simple constipation arising from a low fibre, low fluid diet.

Mode of action

These are also referred to as fibre-like laxatives and they will increase the faecal bulk by directly increasing the volume of faecal material, which stimulates peristalsis. They may add to faecal mass by acting as substrates for the growth of colonic bacteria. Some compounds trap water in the colon by forming a viscous gel. This leads to an increase in the weight of the faeces, softens the faeces and reduces overall transit time.

Contraindications

Intestinal obstruction, atonic colon, and faecal impaction.

Adverse effects

Flatulence and abdominal distention.

Nursing Points

These preparations should be taken with a glass of water. They should be consumed immediately as a 'jelly-like' substance is formed. They should not be taken before going to bed in order to reduce the risk of obstruction.

Osmotic laxatives and rectal preparations:

- Lactulose
- Lactitol
- Macrogol (Movicol®)
- Magnesium hydroxide
- Phosphate enema
- Sodium citrate enemas (Micolette®, Micralax®, Relaxit®)

Mode of action

These products, all of which are poorly absorbed from the intestine, retain fluid in the large intestine by osmosis, or by changing the pattern of water distribution in the faeces. The retention of fluid in the lumen then causes intestinal distention and eventual peristalsis. Osmotic laxatives and rectal preparations include the following.

Lactulose is a synthetic disaccharide or sugar, which is unaffected by the disaccharidase enzyme in the small intestine, and hence it is not absorbed. Lactulose remains in the intestine and exerts its laxative effect by pulling water into the intestinal lumen. Lactulose undergoes fermentation in the colon and this produces gas and short-chain fatty acids. Ultimately, these will stimulate intestinal motility and increase the growth of bowel flora, both of which accelerate transit time and increase stool weight respectively (Spiller and Farthing, 1994).

Lactulose is used in chronic constipation whilst magnesium preparations, phosphate enemas, and sodium citrate enemas provide a more prompt and complete evacuation.

Contraindications

Lactulose is contraindicated in intestinal obstruction and galactosaemia.

Macrogol should be avoided in patients with intestinal obstruction, paralytic ileus, and severe inflammatory conditions (Crohn's disease, ulcerative colitis, toxic megacolon).

The other products in this group should not be used if intestinal obstruction and other acute gastrointestinal conditions are present.

Adverse effects

Lactulose may cause cramps, flatulence, and general abdominal discomfort.

Macrogol may cause abdominal distention, pain, and nausea.

The other products in this group may induce colic and gastrointestinal irritation.

Nursing Points

Lactulose is best administered with either water or fruit juice and may take 48 h to have any effect. Magnesium hydroxide mixture should be shaken well before use and then taken with a full glass of water. The patient should be informed that it will take 2–4 h to have an effect.

Stimulant laxatives and rectal preparations:

- Dantron (Co-danthramer, Co-danthrusate)
- Senna (Senokot®)
- Bisacodyl
- Glycerol (Glycerin) suppositories
- Sodium picosulfate elixir

Mode of action

These products are also referred to as irritant or contact laxatives. They will increase motility of the large intestine by inducing peristaltic activity. They stimulate the intrinsic nerve plexuses to initiate large propulsive waves. Chronic use of these products may lead to 'melanosis coli' (hyperpigmentation of the colon) and irreversible damage to the nerve plexuses. Spiller (1990) suggests that stimulant laxatives used infrequently, perhaps no more than once a week, at the minimal effective dose are unlikely to cause significant harm.

Codanthramer use has been associated with a carcinogenic risk in rodents and long-term exposure to this drug should be avoided. It may be suitable however for the management of analgesia-induced constipation in the terminally ill, and in the short-term for conditions where defaecation must be free from strain (National Prescribing Centre, 1999).

Stimulant laxatives are particularly used to treat constipation caused by prolonged bed rest, neurologic dysfunction of the colon and constipating drugs.

Contraindications

Senna, bisacodyl, dantron, and sodium picosulfate should all be avoided in intestinal obstruction or undiagnosed abdominal pain. They should preferably be avoided in children and used with caution in pregnancy, as they may stimulate uterine activity. Milder laxatives would be more suitable.

Adverse effects

Senna, bisacodyl, dantron, and sodium picosulfate may all cause griping and abdominal cramps. Bisacodyl suppositories may cause some local irritation to the rectum.

Nursing Points

Senna should be taken with adequate fluid and will have its effect within 8–12 h.

Bisacodyl should be taken after food and not within 1 h of other drugs. It will have an effect in 10–12 h. The effect of the suppository usually occurs in 20–60 min but the suppository must be in contact with the rectal mucosa for the best effect.

Dantron is best taken at bedtime and takes 6–12 h to have an effect.

Glycerol suppositories should be moistened with water and inserted directly into faeces to be effective.

Faecal softeners and lubricants:

Preparations include:

- Docusate sodium (Dioctyl®, Fletchers'Enemette®, Norgalax®)
- Arachis oil retention enema

Mode of action

These products assist mucous in the lubrication of faeces to promote easier passage as well as softening faeces.

In addition, some, such as docusate sodium, also lower the surface tension of the faecal material, which then allows fluid to penetrate and soften the stool. Docusate sodium also possesses some stimulant activity. Liquid paraffin was considered the classical lubricant and stool softener but should no longer be used due to problems which include impaired absorption of fat-soluble vitamins, potential inhalation of oil droplets causing a lipid pneumonia, anal seepage of oil and risk of carcinoma from prolonged use (Crossland, 1980).

Softeners should be used in patients that need to avoid straining during defaecation. For example, after myocardial infarction, surgery or in patients with hernias or ano-rectal problems.

Contraindications

Oral docusate sodium should not be prescribed in intestinal obstruction or patients with nausea, vomiting, and abdominal pain. Rectal preparations should be avoided in patients with haemorrhoids and anal fissure.

Adverse effects

Oral docusate sodium may cause nausea, anorexia, and cramps.

Nursing Points

Better absorption occurs when oral docusate sodium is taken alone and not within an hour of other drugs. Adequate water should be consumed at the same time. A laxative effect is seen in 1–2 days.

The arachis oil enema is likely to be most effective if warmed and retained by the patient for as long as possible.

Choice of Laxative or Rectal Preparation

General principles

If the constipation appears to be simple or functional and is not likely to be secondary to underlying disease, then management should not require medical intervention.

Several preparations are available from which the nurse prescriber may select. For many patients bulk-forming drugs should be the first choice, as these mimic the natural action of food on the intestine and can be used over a longer period of time, if required. For patients in whom straining is potentially harmful or painful, faecal softeners are the agents of choice. A short course of a stimulant laxative may be of use if patients do not respond to bulk-forming drugs or appear to have more advanced constipation. Severe constipation and faecal impaction may only respond initially to the use of suppositories or enemas. Where possible, manual evacuation of the rectum should be avoided. This may be very distressing, painful, and potentially dangerous for the patient. Oral laxatives are contraindicated when impaction is present but may be prescribed when the faecal mass has been removed. A bulk-forming agent daily or another laxative once or twice weekly may be necessary if the patient fails to respond to dietary and other non-pharmacological measures.

An informed decision about the choice of product should be made following consideration of the patient's physical condition and psycho-social factors.

Prescribing in children

Few paediatricians appear to be in favour of laxatives and enemas for children and regular dosing is discouraged unless specifically prescribed by a physician. Primary constipation should be managed by dietary adjustments and these will depend on the age of the child. In addition, plenty of fluid, exercise, a suitable toileting environment and provision of adequate time for defaecation are essential. If dietary modification fails to relieve the problem then a single glycerol suppository may provide a satisfactory response (Nathan, 1996). Stool softeners may be given to older children but stimulant laxatives should be avoided.

Evaluation of treatment

Successful treatment should be reinforced by patient education in order to prevent recurrence. This should include information about life-style changes and not buying over-the-counter laxatives. Both repeat prescriptions from the nurse prescriber and purchases of laxatives by the patient should be avoided. Both will increase the chances of laxative abuse, which ultimately may perpetuate the constipation.

Most patients that require continued treatment will benefit from a bulk-forming laxative. Some patients will require a laxative prescription indefinitely, for example, those receiving opiate medication. Unresolved constipation should be followed up by further assessment from the patient's general practitioner in case of the presence of other pathology.

References

AAP: American Academy of Pediatrics (1996). Practice parameter: the management of acute gastroenteritis in young children. *Pediatrics* 97: 424–435.

Avery ME, Snyder JD (1990). Oral therapy for acute diarrhoea. The underused simple solution. *New England Journal of Medicine* 323: 891–894.

Bennet RG, Greenough WB (1987). Diarrhoea: a ubiquitous disease in older persons. *Clinical report on aging (the American Geriatric Society)* 1: 1–9.

Brooks GF, Butel JS, Ornston LN, Jawetz E, Melnick JL, Adelberg EA (1991). *Medical Microbiology* (19th edn). Norwalk: Appleton and Lange.

Crossland J (1980). *Lewis's Pharmacology* (5th edn). Edinburgh: Churchill Livingstone.

DoH (1991). Report on Health and Social Subjects 41. Dietary Reference Values for Food Energy and Nutrients for the United Kingdom. London: HMSO.

DoH (2000). *Referral Guidelines for Suspected Cancer*. Department of Health.

DTB (1996). The medical management of gastro-oesophageal reflux. *Drugs and Therapeutics Bulletin* 34(1): 1–4.

Farthing M, Feldman R, Finch R, Fox R, Leen C, Mandal B, Moss P, Nathwani D, Nye F, Percival A, Read R, Ritchie L, Todd WTA, Wood M (1996). The management of infectivegastroenteritis in adults. A consensus statement by an expert panel convened by the British Society for the Study of Infection. *Journal of Infection* 33: 143–152.

Galbraith A, Bullock S, Manias E, Hunt B, Richards A (1999). *Fundamentals of Pharmacology*. Harlow: Addison Wesley Longman.

Griffin GE, Sissons JGP, Chiodini PL, Mitchell DM (1999). Diseases due to infection. In: Haslett C, Chilvers ER, Hunter JAA, Boon NA (eds). *Davidson's Principles and Practice of Medicine*. Edinburgh: Churchill Livingstone.

Hardy C, Trueman I, MacKown A (2001). All mouth and no action. *Journal of Community Nursing* 15(7): 4–8.

Kumar P, Clark M (1998). Gastroenterology. In: Kumar P, Clark M (eds). Clinical Medicine (4th edn). *Clinical Medicine*. Edinburgh: WB Saunders.

Lehner T (2000). The mouth and salivary glands. In: Ledingham JGG, Warrell DA (eds). *Concise Oxford Textbook of Medicine*. Oxford: Oxford University Press.

Li Wan Po A, Li Wan Po G (1992). *OTC Medications: Symptoms and Treatments of Common Illnesses*. Oxford: Blackwell Scientific Publications.

McCance KL, Huether SE (1994). *Pathophysiology: The Biologic Basis of Disease in Adults and Children* (2nd edn). St. Louis: Mosby.

Mallet J, Bailey C (1996). *The Royal Marsden NHS Trust Manual of Clinical Nursing Procedures* (4th edn). Oxford: Blackwell Science.

Martini FH (2001). *Fundamentals of Anatomy and Physiology* (5th edn). Upper Saddle River: Prentice Hall.

Mims CA, Playfair JHL, Roitt IM, Wakelin D, Williams R, Anderson RM (1993). *Medical Microbiology*. St Louis: Mosby.

Murphy MS (1998). Guidelines for managing acute gastroenteritis based on a systemic review of published research. *Archives of Disease in Childhood* 79: 279–284.

Nathan A (1996). Laxatives. *The Pharmaceutical Journal* 257: 52–55.

Nathan A (1997). Anthelmintics. *The Pharmaceutical Journal* 258: 770–771.

National Prescribing Centre (1999). Prescribing laxatives. *Prescribing Factsheet 15*. National Prescribing Centre.

Porter S, Scully C (2000). Aphthous ulcers: recurrent. *Clinical Evidence* 4: 746–752.

Porth C (1998). *Pathophysiology: concepts of altered health states* (5th edn). Philadelphia: Lippincott.

Spiller RC (1990). Management of constipation – when fibre fails. *British Medical Journal* 300: 1064–1065.

Spiller RC, Farthing MJG (1994). *Diarrhoea and Constipation*. London: Science Press.

Travis SPL, Taylor RH, Misiewicz JJ (1998). *Gastroenterology* (2nd edn). Oxford: Blackwell Science.

Turner G (1996). Oral care (RCN Continuing Education). *Nursing Standard* 10(28): 51–56.

Twycross R (2000). Palliative care: anorexia, cachexia, nausea and vomiting. *Medicine* 28: 7–12.

Chapter 5

Preparations for Problems and Minor Ailments of the Respiratory System

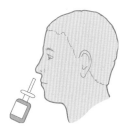

The Respiratory Tract

The respiratory tract can be divided into an upper and lower respiratory system. The upper system consists of the nose, nasal cavity, and pharynx. The lower system consists of the larynx (voice box), trachea (windpipe), bronchi, bronchioles, and alveoli (Martini, 2000).

The nose and nasal cavity

The nose is the first part of the respiratory tract. Within the nose are two nasal passages. The nasal passages have a rich blood supply, which keeps them warm, and many secretory cells, which keep the passages moist. Therefore, the air is both warmed and humidified prior to entering the respiratory tract. Nasal hair and cilia also remove dust particles, which may be present in the air.

The pharynx

This is a tube consisting primarily of muscle and contains the adenoids and tonsils. The tonsils comprise of lymphoid tissue lying below the surface epithelium. The adenoids (nasopharyngeal tonsils), prominent in the young, are uppermost. The palatine tonsils are situated at the back of the oral cavity, and the lingual tonsils are at the base of the tongue. Lymphoid tissue protects the body against infection by filtering out invading micro-organisms. The pharynx leads from the oral cavity and nose to the larynx and the oesophagus.

The larynx

The larynx is a cartilaginous box. It contains the epiglottis (which prevents food from entering the respiratory passageway) and the vocal cords.

Figure 5.1 – The respiratory system

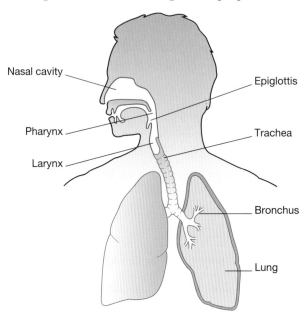

Nasal cavity

Epiglottis

Pharynx

Trachea

Larynx

Bronchus

Lung

The trachea

The trachea is a tough, flexible tube kept open by a number of C-shaped cartilages. Like the nasal cavity, it contains secretory cells.

The bronchi

The trachea branches and divides into the right and left bronchi. Like the trachea, the bronchi are composed of cartilaginous C-shaped rings. The right bronchus supplies the right lung and the left bronchus supplies the left lung (Figure 5.1).

The Lungs

Each lung is cone shaped and divided into distinct lobes. The right lung has three lobes, the left lung has two lobes.

Bronchi

The left and right bronchi divide to form smaller passageways. This is called the bronchiole tree.

Bronchioles

Each bronchus divides several times giving rise to multiple bronchioles. These branch further into very fine conducting branches called terminal bronchioles and finally, into even finer respiratory bronchioles.

Figure 5.2 – Terminal airways and alveoli

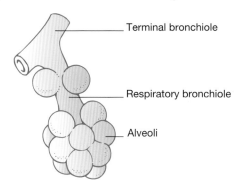

Terminal bronchiole

Respiratory bronchiole

Alveoli

Alveoli

The respiratory bronchioles are connected to the alveoli. Each alveolus is less than the size of a full stop and covered in blood capillaries. Approximately 150 million alveoli are contained within each lung and they give the lung a spongy appearance. Gas exchange occurs at the alveoli (Figure 5.2).

Acute nasopharyngitis (coryza or the common cold)

Acute nasopharyngitis or the common cold is the most frequently occurring upper respiratory disorder. It is extremely contagious. The virus causing acute nasopharyngitis is spread in droplets when sneezing and coughing, and by direct contact. The invading micro-organism is trapped in mucus produced in the upper respiratory tract. The immunological response of the host causes a local inflammatory reaction. The nasal passages become red and swollen, and there is secretion of a clear watery fluid and nasal congestion accompanied by coughing and sneezing. The individual may also experience a low grade fever and aching muscles. Symptoms can persist from a couple of days or for up to 2 weeks. Preparations for pain relief may be prescribed for acute nasopharyngitis. For a list of these preparations, mode of action, contraindications, adverse effects and nursing points *see* Chapter 3.

Acute sore throat (pharyngitis, laryngitis or tonsillitis)

Inflammation of the oropharynx is called pharyngitis. It is usually viral in origin but it can also be caused by bacteria. The common causative bacteria is *Group A beta-haemolytic streptococcus* (LeMone and Burke, 1996). Tonsilitis is an acute inflammation of the tonsils. Tonsilitis can be viral in origin, however, it is frequently due to streptococcal infections (LeMone and Burke, 1996). Laryngitis presents as inflammation of the larynx. It can occur in individuals with respiratory infections such as bronchitis and pneumonia. The lining of the larynx becomes inflamed, there may be oedema of the vocal cords, and a hoarseness of the voice.

Pain relief may be prescribed for individuals suffering from an acute sore throat (*see* Chapter 3). Antibiotics are recommended if there is marked systemic upset;

peritonsillar cellulitis, a history of rheumatic fever; or an increased risk from an acute infection, however these must be prescribed by a doctor (National Institute for Clinical Excellence (NICE) 2000).

Nursing Points

It is important to provide reassurance to the patient with an acute sore throat. Pain relief may be all that is necessary and a gargle may offer relief (although there is little research to support this). Medical advice should be sought if there is a suspected peritonsillar abscess, epiglottitis (examination of the throat should not be undertaken however, drooling of saliva will indicate this condition) (MCA, 2001), or if the voice has been hoarse for 3 weeks or more (DoH, 2000).

Allergic rhinitis

Allergic rhinitis occurs as a result of hypersensitivity to allergens, e.g. pollen. The pollen activates inflammatory cells (mast cells) in the respiratory tract. These cells release histamine and other inflammatory substances (or mediators). Histamine acts on H_1 receptors in the skin, blood vessels, nasal passages, and airways. It also acts on H_2 receptors in the lining of the stomach, lacrimal, and salivary glands (Henry, 2001). This causes vasodilation and increased capillary permeability. Mucous membranes become swollen and congested resulting in sneezing with a watery discharge, watery itchy eyes, and narrowing of the airways.

If possible, the allergen should be avoided. Drug treatment includes topical nasal corticosteroids, oral and topical antihistamines.

Preparations for the treatment of allergic rhinitis:

- Acrivastine capsules 8 mg capsules (Semprex®, Benadryl Allergy Relief®)
- Alimemazine tartrate syrup 7.5 mg/5 ml (Vellergan®)
- Alimemazine tartrate tablets 10 mg (Vellergan®)
- Azelastine hydrochloride aqueous nasal spray 140 μg per spray (Rhinolast®)
- Cetirizine hydrochloride oral solution 5 mg/5 ml (Zirtek®)
- Cetirizine hydrochloride tablets 10 mg (Zirtek®)
- Fexofenadine hydrochloride tablets 120 mg (Telfast® 120)
- Levocabastine 0.05% hydrochloride aqueous nasal spray (Levostin®)
- Loratadine syrup 5 mg/5 ml (Clarityn®)
- Loratadine tablets 10 mg (Clarityn®)
- Beclometasone diproprionate aqueous nasal spray 50 μg per spray (Beconase®)
- Betamethasone sodium phosphate drops 0.1% (Betnesol®, Vista-Methasone®)

- Budesonide nasal spray 100 μg per spray (Rhinocort Aqua®)
- Dexamethasone isonicotinate 20 μg and tramazoline hydrochloride 120 μg per spray (Dexa-Rhinaspray Duo®)
- Flunisolide aqueous nasal spray 25 μg per spray (Syntaris®)
- Fluticasone proprionate aqueous nasal spray 50 μg per spray (Flixonase®)
- Mometasone Furoate aqueous nasal spray 50 μg per spray (Nasonex®)
- Triamcinolone acetonide aqueous nasal spray 55 μg per spray (Nasocort®)

Mode of action

- *Antihistamines* – As mentioned above, histamine has an important role in the allergic response. Antihistamines are widely used in allergic reactions. They work by blocking H_1 receptors and so the action of histamine. The modes of action of corticosteroids are discussed in Chapter 6.

Adverse effects

Antihistamines cross the blood brain barrier producing a sedative effect.

Acrivastine, cetirizine, fexofenadine, and loratadine, are newer antihistamines and penetrate the blood-brain barrier to a lesser extent. Therefore, they are less likely to cause drowsiness, which is the main adverse effect of antihistamines. However, individuals should be warned about the sedatory properties of these preparations and should avoid alcohol, as this will accentuate the depressant effect of these drugs. They should also be advised not to drive.

Levocabastine 0.05% hydrochloride aqueous nasal spray (Levostin®). The systemic absorption of this drug is minimal and so central effects are avoided. However, irritation to the mucosal surface has been reported (Galbraith *et al.*, 1999).

Azelastine hydrochloride aqueous nasal spray 140 μg per spray (Rhinolast®). Adverse effects of this preparation include irritation of the nasal mucosa and taste disturbances.

The adverse effects produced by corticosteroids are outlined in Chapter 6. However, these adverse effects are greatly reduced when these preparations are administered nasally. Systemic absorption may occur if high doses are given over a long period of time. Local adverse effects that may be experienced include disturbances of smell and taste and irritation of the nose and throat. If there is a nasal infection, intranasal corticosteroids should be avoided (MeReC, 1998).

Ipratropium bromide nasal spray 21 μg metered dose (Rinatec®). This preparation is an anticholinergic bronchodilator. It can be prescribed as a nasal spray in an allergic reaction. Adverse effects are rare, the most common being a dry mouth or throat.

Nursing Points

Symptoms of allergic rhinitis include sneezing, rhinorrhoea, and nasal blockage. The eyes, nose, and palate are itchy and the patient may feel lethargic (MeReC, 1998). Confirmation of diagnosis might be aided by a skin prick test (MeReC, 1998). Patients should avoid exposure to pollen by spending time indoors when the pollen count is high and ensuring windows and doors are closed. Treatment is dependent upon symptoms and whether patients prefer topical or oral preparations. The following regime is recommended by the International Rhinitis Management Working Group (Lund *et al.*, 1994).

Mild disease with occasional symptoms

If symptomatic administer a rapid onset oral antihistamine or, a topical antihistamine or cromoglycate to eyes and nose.

Moderate disease with prominent nasal symptoms

Intranasal corticosteroid and topical antihistamines or cromoglycate to the eyes if necessary.

Moderate disease and prominent eye symptoms

Oral antihistamines or, intranasal steroid and topical cromoglycate to the eyes.

Watery rhinorrhoea

The addition of intranasal ipratropium to existing therapy.

The different treatments available vary with regards to their ability to relieve certain symptoms. The symptoms and the most effective treatments have been described by Lund *et al.*, 1994 and include the following:

Nasal itching and sneezing

- Topical corticosteroids
- Oral antihistamines
- Oral corticosteroids (can only be prescribed by a doctor)
- Sodium cromoglycate (marginally effective)

Rhinorrhoea

- Topical corticosteroids
- Ipratropium bromide
- Oral corticosteroids
- Oral antihistamines (moderately effective)
- Sodium cromoglycate (marginally effective)

Nasal blockage

- Oral corticosteroids
- Topical decongestants
- Topical corticosteroids (moderately effective)

Impaired smell

- Oral corticosteroids (moderately effective)
- Topical corticosteroids (marginally effective)

Lund *et al.*, 1994 also suggests that the following must be considered if the treatment applied is not effective:

- Patient compliance
- Whether nasal sprays are being used correctly
- Alternative treatment, e.g. a short course of oral steroids. In this situation, medical advice must be sought

Topical corticosteroids may take several weeks before they produce an effect and therefore, antihistamines may be used during this intermediate period. If the patient has previously experienced allergic rhinitis, treatment should be commenced before the symptoms of the condition appear. Choice of nasal steroid depends on cost and patient preference, as there is a lack of evidence supporting the use of one treatment over another.

Choice of antihistamine also should be based on response and patient preference. A short acting preparation to relieve intermittent symptoms may be preferred over a product which provides longer term relief.

Patients suffering from acute rhinitis must be encouraged to use the preparations as outlined in the product literature. It is important that products that do not produce an immediate effect are used regularly.

Acute sinusitis

Sinusitis in an infection affecting the mucous membranes of the paranasal sinuses (Figure 5.3). This condition usually follows an upper respiratory tract infection and is usually caused by bacteria. Mucus secretions collect in the sinus cavity providing a medium for bacterial growth. As the nasal and sinus mucous membranes are continuous the infection easily spreads. An inflammatory response occurs causing

Figure 5.3 – Sinuses (frontal view)

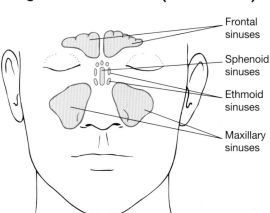

Frontal sinuses

Sphenoid sinuses

Ethmoid sinuses

Maxillary sinuses

increased swelling and pressure. Symptoms include, pain, headache, tenderness, and general malaise. Pain relief (*see* Chapter 3) is usually all that is required as the condition settles spontaneously within a few days. However, antibiotics may be required but must be prescribed by a doctor.

Excessive respiratory secretions

Excessive respiratory secretions may arise in patients with advanced cancer. Preparations are available which reduce these secretions and so prevent coughing or rattling breathing.

Preparations for the management of excessive respiratory secretions:

- Hyoscine hydrobromide 400–600 µg/ml injection (Hyoscine non-proprietary)
- Hyoscine hydrobromide transdermal patch 1 mg hyoscine released/72 h (Scopoderm TTS)
- Hyoscine butylbromide 20 mg/ml injection (Buscopan)

Adverse effects

The above preparations of hyoscine produce a number of adverse effects including tachycardia, drowsiness, dry mouth, blurred vision, constipation and difficulty in passing urine.

References

DoH (2000). *Referral Guidelines for Suspected cancer*. DoH.

Galbraith A, Bullock S, Manias E, Hunt B, Richards A (1999). *Fundamentals of Pharmacology*. UK: Addison Wesley Longman Ltd.

Henry JA (2001). *The British Medical Association Concise Guide to Medicines and Drugs*. London: Dorling Kindersley.

LeMone P, Burke K (1996). *Medical Surgical Nursing*. California: Addison-Wesley.

Lund VJ, Aaronson D, *et al.* (1994) International consensus report on the diagnosis and management of rhinitis. *Allergy* 49(suppl 19): 1–34.

Martini FH (2000): *Fundamentals of Anatomy and Physiology* (5th edn). New Jersey: Prentice Hall International.

MCA (2001). Extended Prescribing of Prescription Only Medicines By Independent Nurse Prescribers. London: MCA.

MeReC (1998). Treatment of seasonal allergic rhinitis (hay fever). Issue No. 47, 183–186. *Medicines Resource Independent Drug Information in Association with the MeReC*. Bulletin produced by the National Prescribing Centre, Liverpool.

NICE (2000). Referral practice: a guide to appropriate referral from general to specialist services. http://www.nice.org.uk

Chapter 6

Preparations for Minor Injuries and Minor Ailments of the Skin

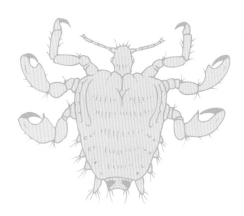

A number of products are available in the NPEF for nurses to prescribe in conditions that affect the skin. This chapter commences with a brief description of the anatomy and physiology of the skin, the physiology of wound healing, and the role of wound dressings in wound healing. A number of conditions that affect the integumentary system and their treatment and management are then examined.

The Skin

The skin is the largest of the body's organs. It has a vast surface area, which spans approximately 2 square metres and accounts for roughly 16% of an individual's total body weight.

The skin (Figure 6.1) is composed of two major layers of tissue the outer epidermis, and the inner dermis. It also has a number of accessory structures including hair, nails, sweat glands, and sebaceous glands. These structures, although located in the dermis, protrude through the epidermis to the skin surface.

The skin has a number of functions (Martini, 2000). These include:

- Protection of underlying organs and tissues.
- Excretion of waste products, salts, and water.
- Maintenance of normal body temperature.
- Storage of nutrients.
- Detection of stimuli such as temperature, and the relay of this information to the nervous system.

Figure 6.1 – Structure of the skin

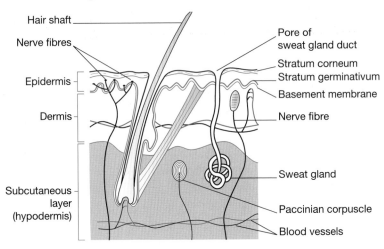

Labels: Hair shaft, Nerve fibres, Epidermis, Dermis, Subcutaneous layer (hypodermis), Pore of sweat gland duct, Stratum corneum, Stratum germinativum, Basement membrane, Nerve fibre, Sweat gland, Paccinian corpuscle, Blood vessels

Epidermis

The skin is persistently subjected to mechanical injury. The epidermis provides protection, and also prevents micro-organisms from entering the body. It is comprised of a number of layers. The innermost layer of the epidermis is called the stratum germinativum, and the outermost layer, the stratum corneum. The stratum germinativum is attached to a basement membrane which separates the dermis from the epidermis.

The stratum germinativum is composed of many germinative or basal cells, the division of which replace the cells shed at the epithelial surface. As these germinative cells move towards the skin surface, their structure, and activity changes. Whilst still at the basal layer, they begin forming a protein called keratin. The formation of this protein is continued as they move towards the skin's surface. Eventually, as the cells reach the stratum corneum, approximately 15–30 days later, they are like flattened bags of protein, and their intracellular organelles have disappeared.

Before they are lost from the stratum corneum, these cells remain in this layer for a further 2 weeks. This provides the underlying tissue with a protective barrier of cells, which although dead, are exceedingly durable. The stratum corneum is the major barrier to the loss of water from the body. It has two actions, which restrain the movement of water, and limit the loss of water from the skin's surface. Firstly, the matrix in which the cells of the stratum corneum are embedded is rich in lipid. This substance is almost impenetrable to water and therefore makes it extremely difficult for water molecules to move out of the epidermal cell. Secondly, protein inside the epidermal cells attracts, and holds on to water molecules. As a consequence of these actions, the surface of the skin is therefore normally dry, with very little water lost and so is, therefore, unsuitable for the growth of many micro-organisms. Although water-resistant, the stratum corneum is not waterproof.

Interstitial fluid gradually penetrates this layer of tissue to be evaporated from the surface into the surrounding air. Approximately 500 ml is lost from the body each day in this way.

Dermis

The dermis is comprised of a network of two types of protein. These proteins are collagen and elastin. The collagen fibres provide strength to the skin. The elastin gives the skin its flexibility. The dermis is also comprised of a network of blood vessels, and a number of other structures. These include, sweat glands which are found all over the skin and secrete a dilute salt solution onto the skin's surface sebaceous glands, found everywhere in the body except non-hairy areas, and which secrete sebum containing a mixture of lipids, sensory receptors, and defence cells.

There are variations in the structure of the skin in relation to age, environment, and ethnic origin. The skin also varies between different parts of the body. For example, non-hairy (glabrous) skin, e.g. on the palms of hands and soles of feet, has an extremely thick epidermis and numerous sensory receptors. The skin with hair follicles, hairy skin, e.g. on the scalp, has a thin epidermis and many sebaceous glands.

The Physiology of Wound Healing

During wounding, there is a breakdown in these protective functions. For example, micro-organisms are able to enter the deeper tissues of the body and cause infection. In burn injuries, large areas of the skin's surface may be damaged to such an extent that fluid loss may become life threatening.

Wounds can be classified by the layers of tissue involved. In superficial wounds, only the epidermis is effected. In partial thickness wounds, injury extends as far as the dermis. Wounds that involve the subcutaneous fat or deeper layers, are classified as full thickness wounds.

Several causes of wounding have been identified by Dealey (1994) and described as those arising through

- trauma (i.e. mechanical, chemical, or physical)
- surgery
- ischaemia (e.g. arterial leg ulcer)
- pressure (e.g. pressure sore)

Incision wounds, closed by suturing, require only the formation of a small quantity of new tissue. This is called healing by primary intention and is accomplished within several days. However, in wounds caused by trauma where there is tissue loss, the formation of new tissue is essential. This new tissue fills the wound and is then covered by epithelium. This is called healing by secondary intention and can take weeks or months.

Regardless of the nature of the tissue damage, the process of healing occurs in three overlapping phases

- Inflammation
- Proliferation
- Maturation

Inflammation

Following tissue damage, bleeding generally occurs. A network of molecules, produced by fibrinogen, bring the wound edges in loose approximation. Fibrin (an insoluble protein which forms the basic framework of a blood clot) and other proteins dry at the surface, and a scab is formed. This prevents further fluid loss and bacterial invasion. Meanwhile, serum proteins and white cells are leaked from blood vessels surrounding the wound. This accumulation of fluid in the tissue gives rise to the signs of inflammation, i.e. swelling, heat, redness, and pain, and occurs within minutes of the injury. Following this, neutrophils and macrophages move into the damaged tissue to remove debris and ingest bacteria.

Proliferation

Following the inflammatory phase, tissue proliferation takes place. This phase involves:

- The formation of a network of new blood vessels in a collagen rich matrix, i.e. granulation, and the appearance of strands of collagen in the body of the wound.
- Contraction of the wound which minimises its size.
- Epithelialisation, which involves the epithelial cells on the wound surface turning down over the edge of the underlying dermis and growing under the dried scab (Figure 6.2).

Maturation

During the final stage of healing, the wound becomes less vascularised, as there is a reduction in the need to bring blood cells to the wound site. The wound is also strengthened by the rearrangement of collagen fibres and the scar tissue is gradually remodelled, becoming comparable to normal tissue.

Wound Assessment

Good wound management requires an accurate assessment, so that the best possible conditions for healing can be provided. The assessment must take into consideration the patient's general condition, their environment and social circumstances, as well as the wound itself.

A wound assessment should include the following (Dunford, 1997):

- The position and size of the wound
- The tissue type (e.g. sloughy or necrotic)
- The amount of exudate
- The presence or absence of infection
- The presence or absence of pain
- The possibility of a sinus

Figure 6.2 – Stages in skin regeneration following injury

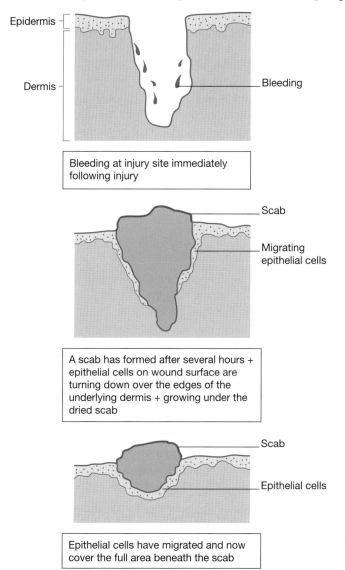

Epidermis

Dermis

Bleeding

Bleeding at injury site immediately following injury

Scab

Migrating epithelial cells

A scab has formed after several hours + epithelial cells on wound surface are turning down over the edges of the underlying dermis + growing under the dried scab

Scab

Epithelial cells

Epithelial cells have migrated and now cover the full area beneath the scab

Thomas (1990) has described a simple wound classification system, representing both the different types of wound, and the stages of healing through which a single wound may pass. This classification is as follows:

- Black and necrotic – covered with a hard, dry, black necrotic layer
- Yellow and sloughy – covered (or filled) with a soft yellow slough
- Clean with significant tissue loss (granulating)
- Clean and superficial (epithelialising)

The Function of a Wound Dressing

Wound dressings are available in a wide range of physical forms with a variety of differing properties. There is no single dressing suitable for all types of wounds, and often a number of dressing types will need to be used during the healing of a single wound. It is therefore important to have an understanding of the functions of each dressing type.

Dressings may perform one or more of the functions listed below

- The maintenance of high humidity at the wound/dressing interface. This speeds up the epithelialisation process, reduces pain and breaks down necrotic tissue.
- The removal of excess exudate thus preventing the maceration of tissue.
- Gaseous exchange, which is thought to be of benefit during some stages of the healing process.
- The provision of thermal insulation. A constant temperature of 37°C promotes both macrophage and mitotic activity during granulation and epithelialisation.
- Impermeability to bacteria. Preventing airborne organisms, and organisms on the surface of the skin from entering the wound.
- Freedom from particles and toxic wound contaminants. Older dressings such as gauze tissue or gamgee, shed particles into the wound, renewing or prolonging the inflammatory process. Modern wound management products do not cause this problem.
- Removal without causing trauma. Dressings, which have adhered to the wounds surface will, on removal, disrupt tissue, and delay healing.

(See Dealey, 1994 for a fuller discussion of the above points)

Prior to the selection of a dressing, it is essential to determine what the wound requires to promote healing. The requirements of the wound, e.g. promotion of debridement, granulation, or epithelialisation, can then be compared with the properties of each of the available dressings.

The functions of a dressing during these various stages of healing have been identified (Thomas, 1990). See Table 6.1.

For wounds that require an external absorbent protective dressing, a number of absorbent cottons, lints, and gauzes are available. Primary dressings for clean, low exudate wounds include Perforated Film Absorbent Dressings, e.g. Melolin®.

Vapour-permeable film dressings, permeable to water vapour, oxygen and other gases (but not to water or bacteria), are commonly used to isolate an area, e.g. a pressure sore, from maceration and friction. Film dressings include, Opsite Flexigrid®, Tegaderm®, and Bioclusive®.

Dressings suitable for clean wounds with a medium to high exudate include Paraffin gauze dressing, and Knitted Varicose Primary Dressings. These dressings are non-adherent to the wound, have a superimposed absorbent pad, and so are effective on ulcerative and other granulating wounds.

Table 6.1 – The functions of a wound dressing

Wound type	Dressing function
Dry, necrotic wounds	Moisture retention
Slough-covered wounds	Moisture retention
	Fluid absorption
	Odour absorption*
	Antimicrobial properties*
Clean, exuding wounds	Fluid absorption
(granulating)	Odour absorption*
	Antimicrobial properties*
	Thermal insulation
Dry, low exudate	Moisture retention
wounds (epithelialising)	Low adherence
	Thermal insulation

*Not always required

The cells of the dermis and the deeper layers of the epidermis are normally bathed in tissue fluid. If damage to the skin occurs, these tissues dry out. A wound that is exposed to the atmosphere will normally form a scab of cellular debris and protein. However, by covering the wound with an occlusive dressing, a moist atmosphere is maintained and the formation of a scab prevented. It has been shown by Winter (1962) that crusted wounds epithelialise more slowly than a wound that has been covered. Occlusive and semi-occlusive dressings available include, alginates, hydrocolloids, hydrogels, and foam dressings. These products and their uses are described below.

Hydrocolloids

Hydrocolloid dressings are made from cellulose, gelatin, and pectins and have a backing of polyurethane film or foam. A number of these products are available as a paste, and others have a border ensuring greater adhesion. When placed in contact with wound exudate, these dressings absorb water and swell to form a gel. This gel forms a moist environment under the dressing and so promotes wound healing. Examples of hydrocolloids include:

- Comfeel®
- Granuflex®
- Tegasorb®

Indications for use

Hydrocolloid dressings should be used on granulating wounds, which have low to moderate exudate. This includes pressure sores, leg ulcers, surgical wounds, and minor burns. They can also be used effectively in the management of blisters, and to facilitate rehydration and autolytic debridement of dry, sloughy or necrotic wounds. The barrier properties of these products prevent the spread of micro-organisms.

Contraindications

Hydrocolloid dressings are not suitable for infected wounds. Heavy exudate leads to frequent dressing changes. These dressings should also be avoided in patients who have a sensitivity to the hydrocolloid or its constituents.

Nursing Points

The choice of hydrocolloid will depend on the condition of the wound, and the individual environmental and social needs of the patient. Hydrocolloids come in a variety of sizes, some being more absorbent than others. All hydrocolloids are impermeable to water, and therefore, can remain in place during showering or bathing. Secondary dressings are unnecessary.

Adhesion of some of these dressings can be a problem with dressing edges rolling off. This can be prevented in a number of ways (Bux, 1996)

- Choose a dressing that allows a minimum overlap of 2cm from the margin of the wound.
- Cover the dressing with an adhesive retention sheet if the product is likely to become disturbed by movement.
- Warm the dressing between the hands to make it more pliable (whilst maintaining asepsis).
- Stop the patient mobilising or putting weight on the dressing for 20 min following application. This allows the adhesive to take full effect.

Ideally these dressings should be left in place for 4–5 days. However, if an infection is present, they will need to be changed more frequently, so that the wound site can be checked. Therefore, an alternative dressing may be more appropriate.

Hydrogels

Hydrogels are made from a co-polymer starch and are capable of retaining significant volumes of water. Examples include:

- Intrasite Gel®
- Nu-Gel®
- Purilon Gel®
- Sterigel®

Two types of hydrogels are available

- *Amorphous products* – e.g. Intrasite Gel® have no firm structure and as moisture is absorbed their viscosity is reduced.
- *Sheet hydrogels* – e.g. Geliperm® whose structure is retained as water is absorbed.

Indications for use

When applied, hydrogel dressings either lose or absorb water depending on the state of hydration of the wound. These dressings are used primarily in dry 'sloughy' or necrotic wounds, lightly exuding wounds, and granulating wounds. These products can also be used in the treatment of malodourous fungating wounds, acting as a carrier for metronidazole.

Contraindications

Hydrogel dressings are not suitable for infected or heavily exuding wounds. Some preparations may cause an allergic reaction. If this occurs, the treatment should be stopped. Wounds that are clinically infected with *Pseudomonas* species should not be treated with sheet hydrogels.

Nursing Points

The needs of the patient and the condition of the wound should be assessed prior to the selection of the dressing. When using amorphous products, a thick layer of gel should be applied to the surface of the wound, followed by a secondary dressing. Sheet hydrogels, once applied to the wound, also need to be covered with a secondary dressing. These should then be changed every 3–4 days. When dressings are applied to dry wounds, it is recommended that they are changed daily. In wounds with abundant exudate, perforated plastic film dressing, followed by an absorbent pad, may be used as the secondary dressing. In wounds with low levels of exudate, vapour-permeable adhesive film dressings can be used.

Foam dressings

These dressings take the form of flat foam dressings and include:

- Lyofoam®
- Allevyn®
- Spyrosorb®
- Cavi-Care®
- Allevyn Cavity Wound Dressing®

Each of these dressings are very different with regards to composition, and the management of each varies greatly. However, generally, these products encourage healing by absorbing exudate and maintaining a moist environment. They are not recommended for dry superficial wounds but tend to be used on exuding, granulating wounds. A secondary dressing is not normally required.

Lyofoam®

Lyofoam® can be used on moderately exuding granulating wounds and sloughy wounds, but are unsuitable for dry wounds. Lyofoam C® is suitable for malodorous wounds. These products have a backing, which is adhesive and waterproof. It is important when applying these dressings that they overlap the wound edges by 2–3 cm. This is because the fluid absorbed from the wound travels sideways across the face of the dressing. Lyofoam® dressings should initially be changed each day but as the exudate lessens, they can be left in situ for 7 days.

Allevyn®

This product consists of polyurethane foam bonded to a vapour-permeable polyurethane film. A plastic net covers the surface of the dressing to prevent it from adhering to granulating tissue. The outer layer is bacteria and waterproof. Allevyn® dressings should be used to treat light to moderately exuding wounds. They can be left on a clean non-infected wound for 3–4 days. However, if exudate is copious they will require changing more frequently.

Spyrosorb®

This layered polyurethane foam film dressing is an absorbent vapour-permeable dressing, which can be used to dress granulating wounds with light to moderate exudate. These products should not be used on wounds that are clinically infected. Dressings require changing when wound exudate is within 1 cm of the edges of the dressing or, after they have been in situ for between 5 and 7 days.

Cavi-Care®

This product is a soft conforming cavity wound dressing. It should be used in deep cavity wounds that are granulating, and broad excision wounds such as pilonidal sinus excision, peri-anal wounds, perineal wounds, and pressure sores. Cavi-Care® should not be used in wounds that are clinically infected, or in deep narrow wounds. If applied to deep narrow wounds, small pieces of the foam may become left in the wound. Cavi-Care® consists of two separate solutions, that should be mixed thoroughly together, for 15 s immediately before use. The resultant foam is then poured into the wound where it expands to form a 'stent'. This 'stent' should be cleaned daily by soaking in an Aqueous Chlorhexidine solution (0.5%). It is important that it is then rinsed and gently squeezed in tap water to remove traces of the chlorhexidine, which may irritate the wound and surrounding area. Cavi-Care® dressings can be used for a week or longer. However, as the wound gradually decreases in size, this time interval will need to be reduced, as a smaller 'stent' will be required.

Allevyn Cavity Wound Dressing®

Allevyn Cavity Wound Dressing® is for cavity wounds that are producing exudate. It is made of foam chippings in a perforated film. A suitable sized dressing must be placed in situ in the cavity followed by a dressing retention sheet. This can then be held in place by tape.

Alginates

Alginate dressings contain calcium alginate, which is derived from seaweed. These products, in the presence of wound exudate, change from a fibrous structure to a gel, which is believed to facilitate healing. Examples of alginates include:

- Keltogel®
- Kaltostat®
- Sorbsan®
- Tegagen®

Indications for use

Alginate dressings are of little value if applied to dry, or lightly exuding wounds. Their primary use is in the treatment of exuding granulating wounds including leg ulcers, acute surgical wounds, sinuses and other cavity wounds, e.g. pressure sores. Malodorous wounds can also be effectively treated with the alginate Sorbsan®.

Contraindications

Alginate dressings are not the dressing of choice for infected wounds. They are also unsuitable for very dry wounds or wounds covered with hard necrotic tissue. Alginates should not be used with topical antimicrobial or antibiotic agents they may prevent the gelling process from occurring.

Nursing Points

Alginate dressings come in a variety of forms, including flat dressings, rope or ribbon, and extra-absorbent versions with an adhesive backing. A major advantage of these products is that they can be removed without causing pain to the patient.

Alginate dressings vary in both their chemical and physical properties. Therefore, it is essential that prior to the selection of a product, a wound assessment be undertaken. It is important that this assessment takes into consideration both the size and condition of the wound, along with the individual needs of the patient. For example, if the patient's environmental and social situation allows bathing, Kaltoclude® and Sorbsan SA® are waterproof and can be worn whilst in the bath.

Certain alginates will cause maceration and excoriation of surrounding skin. Therefore, particular attention must be paid when applying these products. If using Kaltostat®, the dressing should be cut or folded to fit flat wounds correctly. An important point to remember when applying alginate dressings, is that they must be covered with a secondary dressing to conserve moisture. Failure to do so, will result in the alginate drying out. The selection of the secondary dressing will depend on the quantity of exudate. In situations where exudate is copious, absorbent pads are effective. However, if exudate is minimal, a vapour-permeable film dressing can be used.

Alginates are biodegradable. However, it is important when removing the dressing, that any remaining traces are removed from the wound. Irrigation with 0.9% sodium chloride solution will dissolve Sorbsan® and Kaltogel®. However, Tegagen® and Kaltostat® are less soluble. Therefore, these dressings need to be soaked in 0.9% sodium chloride prior to removal. They can then be removed intact from the wound.

It is possible to leave alginate dressing products in place for 7 days. Although, ideally they should be removed after they have been in situ between 3 and 5 days. In circumstances where wounds have large amounts of exudate, manufacturers recommend that dressings be changed daily. However, if appropriate, secondary dressings are selected, they will absorb the exudate, which will prevent interrupting the moist wound environment. Kaltostat Fortex® sheets are also very effective in heavily exuding wounds. This product has an increased absorbent capacity, which will allow fewer dressing changes. In situations where wounds are infected, daily dressing changes should be considered.

Table 6.2 summarises the different types of wounds and describes the appropriate dressing types.

Table 6.2 – Wound type and appropriate dressing

Wound type	Type of dressing
Dry, necrotic wounds	Hydrocolloids and hydrogels
Slough-covered wounds	Hydrocolloids and hydrogels
Clean, exuding wounds (granulating)	Hydrocolloids, foams, alginates
Clean, dry, low exudate wounds (epithelialising)	Absorbent perforated plastic film-faced dressing
	Vapour-permeable adhesive film dressings
Clean, medium-to-high exudate wounds (epithelialising)	Knitted varicose primary dressing
	Paraffin gauze

Abrasions

A number of terms are used to describe injuries to the skin. The type of wound will dictate the treatment required in order to promote healing. An injury which produces a break in the epithelium is an open wound. Martini (2000) describes an abrasion as an open wound which has arisen as a result of scraping against a solid object. Pain relief may be required for an abrasion (*see* Chapter 3).

Nursing Points

Although bleeding from an abrasion may only be slight, a considerable area is open to infection. The area should therefore be cleaned. It may then be covered with a dressing or, left exposed to the air.

Minor lacerations

A minor laceration is a superficial open wound of the skin resulting from cutting or tearing. It does not involve other structures.

Nursing Points

Treatment involves stopping any bleeding, cleaning, pain relief (*see* Chapter 3) suturing (if necessary), the application of an appropriate dressing, possible tetanus vaccination, and antibiotics if the wound is infected. These must be prescribed by a doctor.

Animal or human bite

Abrasions or small lacerations generally result from an animal or human bite. However, the bite may penetrate the integument, i.e. a puncture wound, and the injury may be quite extensive.

Nursing Points

Medical advice should be sought if the wound is extensive. The treatment for abrasions and lacerations are described above. Co-amoxiclav is recommended for all bites (Drugs and Therapeutic Bulletin (DTB) 1996). For those individuals that are penicillin-sensitive, dog bites should be treated with erythromycin, cat bites with a tetracycline, and human bites with both erythromycin and metronidazole (MCA, 2001). These preparations must be prescribed by a doctor.

Acne

Acne occurs in both males and females at about the time of puberty. It is a disease of the sebaceous glands (Galbraith et al., 1999). Sebaceous glands are found attached to hair follicles in the skin. Sebum, a natural waxy secretion, produced by these glands, normally escapes from the follicle along the hair. If too much sebum is produced, its flow becomes blocked (by debris produced by the skin, or, sebum which has become hardened). This leads to an accumulation of sebum and a spot (acne). If bacteria are trapped beneath this plug of sebum (usually *Propionibacterium acnes*) they can multiply and form blackheads, inflamed spots (papules), pustules (a spot containing pus) and whiteheads. Henry (2001) classifies mild acne as that presenting with blackheads and an occassional pustule. Moderate acne is described as involving large numbers of pustules and papules and, in severe acne, the skin becomes inflamed and cysts (pus enclosed within scar tissue) can be found in the inflamed dermis.

A number of preparations are used to treat acne. These include keratolytics, antimicrobials or retinoids.

Preparations for the treatment of acne:

Antimicrobials
- Oxytetracycline tablets
- Doxycycline capsules or dispersable tablets
- Tetracycline tablets or capsules
- Minocycline tablets or capsules
- Azelic acid 20% cream (Skinoren®)
- Clindamycin phosphate lotion 1% in aqueous basis (Dalacin T®)
- Clindamycin phosphate topical solution 1% in aqueous alcoholic basis (Dalacin T®)
- Erythromycin 2% and 4% in alcoholic gel basis (Eryacne®2, Eryacne®4)
- Erythromycin 2% solution in alcoholic basis (Stiemycin®)
- Erythromycin 40 mg and zinc acetate 12 mg/ml in ethanol solvent (Zineryt®)
- Tetracycline hydrochloride 2.2 mg/ml solution (Topicycline®)

Retinoids

- Adapalene 0.1% cream and gel (Differin®)
- Isotretinoin gel 0.05% (Isotrex®)
- Isotretinoin 0.05% and erythromycin 2% in ethanolic gel (Isotrexin®)
- Tretinoin 0.025% cream, 0.01% and 0.025% gel, 0.025% lotion (Retin-A®)

Keratolytics

- Benzoyl peroxide 5% and erythromycin 3% in an alcoholic basis (Benzamycin®)

The mode of action, contraindications, adverse effects and nursing points for antimicrobials can be found in Chapter 2.

Benzoyl peroxide

Mode of action

Benzoyl peroxide unblocks sebaceous glands by removing the top layer of skin. Inflammation of the blocked follicle is reduced as this preparation also kills the bacteria causing the infection (Henry, 2001).

Caution

Benzoyl peroxide should not be allowed to come into contact with the mouth, mucous membranes or eyes.

Adverse effects

Skin irritation.

Retinoids

Mode of action

Retinoids appear to reduce sebum production and enable the drainage of sebum by causing the epidermal layer to be less cohesive (Hopkins, 1999).

Contraindications

Retinoids should not be applied during pregnancy or, if breast feeding. Tretinoin is contraindicated if an individual has a history of cutaneous epithelioma.

Cautions

These preparations should not be applied when acne covers a large surface area or, if the skin is broken. Exposure to ultra violet light and cosmetic astringents should also be avoided.

Adverse effects

The adverse effects of these preparations include local irritation (Adapalene can sometimes be less irritant), dry skin, and an increased sensitivity to sunlight. During the initial stages of treatment with tretinoin, acne can become exacerbated.

Nursing Points

In mild cases of acne, regular washing and moderate exposure to sunlight or ultraviolet light is normally all that is required. Topical preparations are generally used to treat mild to moderate acne, i.e. benzoyl peroxide, azaleic acid cream, retinoids, and antibiotics. In more severe cases, oral antibiotics might be required.

Boils/carbuncles

Bacterial skin infections develop in the hair follicle. These infections can spread into deeper tissue resulting in a systemic infection which can be life threatening. Folliculitis, furuncles, carbuncles, cellulitis, erysipelas, and impetigo are all bacterial skin infections.

Folliculitis, furuncles, and carbuncles

Bacterial infections of the hair follicle are called folliculitis. *Staphylococcus aureus* is generally the causative micro-organism. The infection develops at the point of follicle opening and penetrates into the follicle causing inflammation and pustules on the surface of the skin. Furuncles or boils can begin as folliculitis but the infection spreads into the dermis by travelling through the follicular wall. A tender cystic nodule develops. Carbuncles involve a group of hair follicles that have become infected. Poor hygiene, poor nutrition, and excessive moisture contribute to these conditions.

These conditions generally resolve spontaneously. Analgesia can be helpful (*see* Chapter 3). If the infection is severe, begins to spread, or there is systemic involvement, antibiotics should be administered (MCA, 2001). These must be prescribed by a doctor.

Burn or scald

A burn is an alteration in the integrity of the skin that results in tissue damage or loss (LeMone and Burke, 1996). Burns can be classified into four categories.

Thermal burns

Thermal burns occur following exposure to flames, steam, and hot liquid.

Chemical burns

When the skin is in contact with either an acidic or basic agent a chemical burn will arise.

Electrical burns

These burns are experienced when the skin is in contact with an electrical current.

Radiation burns

These burns are normally superficial and are associated with sunburn or radiation treatment.

Products in the NPEF enable nurses to provide treatment for minor burns, i.e. thermal or radiation burns. Treatment is as for abrasions (*see* page 104). Oral analgesia will provide pain relief (*see* Chapter 3) and a tetanus vaccination may also need to be given.

Candidiasis of the skin

Candida albicans is the yeast-like, opportunistic fungus that is usually responsible for candida infection of the skin (*see* Chapter 4 for a discussion of this fungus).

Preparations for the treatment of candidiasis of the skin:

- Clotrimazole 1% and betamethasone 0.05% as dipropionate cream (Lotriderm®)
- Clotrimazole 1% and hydrocortisone 1% cream (Canesten HC®)
- Econazole 1% and hydrocortisone 1% cream (Econacort®)
- Ketoconazole 2% cream (Nizoral®)
- Miconazole nitrate 2% and hydrocortisone 1% cream and ointment (Daktacort®)
- Nystatin cream 100,000 units/g, hydrocortisone 0.5%, and chlorhexidine hydrochloride 1%, ointment nystatin 100,000 units/g, hydrocortisone 0.5% and chlorhexidine acetate 1% (Nystaform-HC®)
- Nystatin 100,000 units/g cream and ointment (Nytan®)
- Sulconazole nitrate 1% cream (Exelderm®)
- Hydrocortisone 0.5%, nystatin 100,000 units/g, benzalkonium chloride solution 0.2%, dimeticone '350' 10% cream (Timodine®)

Clotrimazole, Econazole, Ketoconazole, and Miconazole, Sulconazole are all imidazoles. The mode of action, contraindications, adverse effects, and nursing points for these preparations and nystatin are discussed in Chapter 4. These preparations are applied topically in candidiasis skin infections. Systemic adverse effects are rare as drug absorption is only slight. However, they can include a diuretic effect, abdominal cramping and local irritation (Galbraith *et al.*, 1999). Some of these products have been combined with a corticosteroid (hydrocortisone or betamethasone) to help alleviate the inflammation that might accompany a fungal infection. These are compound preparations.

Corticosteroids

Corticosteroid hormones are formed in the cortex of the adrenal glands. Corticosteroids have two effects, i.e. mineralocorticoid or glucocorticoid. Glucocorticoid effects include the maintenance of normal blood sugar levels and they assist the body to recover in times of injury or stress. Mineralocorticoid effects include controlling the balance between the water content and mineral salts in the body. Large amounts of corticosteroids in the body will suppress the activity of the immune system and produce an anti-inflammatory effect. This is the main reason for their therapeutic use.

Mode of action

Corticosteroids act by enzyme inhibition, suppressing the formation of prostaglandin and leukotriene inflammatory mediators. They also decrease histamine release from basophils. Their effect is therefore to suppress the inflammation and allergic/immune responses (Hopkins, 1999).

Adverse effects

Adverse effects occur most frequently if an individual is receiving a potent or high dose of corticosteroid therapy or, if treatment is long-term and systemic. Adverse effects include:

- Hyperglycaemia and diabetes mellitus
- Protein catabolism leading to a loss of bone mass, muscle atrophy, and paper thin skin
- Lipolysis which can lead to an alteration of subcutaneous fat distribution resulting in a 'moon-face' and 'buffalo-hump'
- Increased susceptibility to infection
- Poor wound healing
- Oedema
- Increased blood pressure
- Sodium and water retention
- Hypokalaemia
- Hirsutism
- Allergic reactions
- Increased gastric acidity leading to an exacerbation of peptic ulcers (Galbraith *et al.*, 1999)

Topical corticosteroids are administered to relieve inflammation and itching in skin diseases.

Topical corticosteroids vary with regard to their potency. The following indicates preparation potency:

- Mildly potent
  - Hydrocortisone
- Moderately potent
  - Alclometasone
  - Clobetasone
  - Fluocinonide
  - Fluocortolone
  - Flurandrenolone
  - Halcinonide
- Potent
  - Beclomethasone
  - Betamethasone
  - Diflucortolone
  - Desoxymethasone

- Fluocinonide
- Fluticasone
- Mometasone
- Triamcinolone
- Very potent
    - Halcinonide
    - Clobetasol (Henry, 2001)

Adverse effects

Mild and moderately potent topical corticosteroids are rarely associated with adverse effects. However, care must be taken if products are applied over a large surface, if an occlusive dressing is applied to the area, or, if the skin is damaged, as systemic absorption will be increased. Permanent changes to the skin will occur if potent corticosteroids are used in high concentrations over a prolonged period of time. Thinning of the skin and prominent blood vessels are the most common adverse effects. Therefore, if they are to be applied to the skin on the face, mild corticosteroids should only be prescribed. Rebound erythroderma (reddening of the skin) can occur if a treatment is stopped abruptly (Henry, 2001).

Nursing Points

Topical antifungal treatment is usually all that is necessary to treat skin candidiasis. If there is inflammation, an antifungal preparation combined with a corticosteroid may be of value. Soap and water should be used to clean the skin prior to applying the product to the affected areas. The preparation should be applied once or twice a day. It should be applied evenly but not too thickly using soft, gentle strokes to ensure absorption (carers or nurses should wear gloves). Medical advice should be sought if the skin infection is extensive or, if the patient is immunocompromised. In these circumstances, systemic antifungal treatment may be more appropriate.

Chronic skin ulcer

Pressure sores, also referred to as decubitus ulcers, may present as persistently hyperaemic, blistered, broken or necrotic skin and may extend to underlying structures, including muscle and bone (Cullum et al., 2000). Pressure sores are common at bony prominences, e.g. shoulders, elbows, hips, sacrum, and heels. Risk factors associated with pressure sore development include impaired mobility, poor nutritional status, diabetes, incontinence, reduced fluid intake, oedema and the age of an individual. Basic nursing interventions involve the relief of pressure by regularly repositioning the patient, and the use of an appropriate mattress when the patient is in bed, or special cushions whilst a person is in a chair. Although different dressings are frequently used to treat pressure sores, their effectiveness is unclear (Cullum et al., 2000).

A leg ulcer is the loss of skin on the leg or foot that takes more than 6 weeks to heal (Nelson *et al.*, 2000).

Leg ulcers are commonly associated with venous disease but can be associated with arterial disease. Careful history taking, examination of the patient, and Doppler ultrasound assessment will exclude significant arterial disease. If the Ankle Brachial Pressure Index (ABPI) is greater than 0.8, multilayer compression bandaging is the most safe and effective treatment (Fletcher, 1997; Nelson *et al.*, 2000). The risk of recurrence is also possibly less if compression hosiery is worn following ulcer healing (Nelson *et al.*, 2000). Compression therapy works by providing pressure and support for the superficial vessels. This counteracts the raised capillary pressure and prevents oedema (*see* Chapter 11 for a discussion of compression hosiery).

Doppler assessment

Prior to the application of compression therapy, it is necessary to exclude arterial insufficiency. This is ensured by careful history taking, examination of the patient, and Doppler ultrasound assessment.

Doppler assessment is used to determine the ABPI. This involves taking both the brachial and ankle systolic pressures using a hand-held Doppler probe to detect blood flow. The ABPI is a comparison between the highest pressure at the ankle and the central systolic blood pressure, i.e. the higher of the two brachial pressures (brachial pressures can vary between each arm).

In order that the Doppler assessment is accurate, it must be standardised with regard to equipment, environment, and procedure. The following points must be considered:

- The cuff width should be 40% of the circumference of the midpoint of the limb, or 20% wider than the diameter.
- Bladder length should be twice its width. If the cuff is too narrow, this could result in an inaccurate high reading.
- Probe sizes vary. However, 5–8 MHz is normally used.
- The correct gel, in the correct quantity, should be applied in order that a good signal is heard.
- It must be recorded if the patient cannot lie down. This standardises the procedure and reduces the risk of the reading being falsely low due to exercise.
- Brachial systolic pressure should be measured in both arms and the higher reading recorded.
- The highest reading of at least two pulses on each leg should be recorded.
- Calcification of arteries can cause a false high reading. This can cause problems in individuals with diabetes (Vowden, 1996).

Calculating the ABPI

The patient should be supine and have been resting for 10–20 min prior to the assessment.

Brachial pressure

- Position the cuff around the upper arm.
- Palpate the brachial pulse and apply the ultrasound gel.
- Place Doppler at an angle of 45° and locate the best signal.
- Arterial flow is a pulsating 'woosh.' Venous flow is a nonpulsatile rush.
- If difficulty is experienced in hearing arterial sounds, increasing the Doppler volume, adding more gel, and gently repositioning the probe will help.
- Inflate the cuff until the signal can no longer be heard. Slowly deflate the cuff and record the pressure at which the signal returns. Ensure that the probe is on the line of artery.
- Repeat the procedure for the other arm. Use the highest value to calculate the ABPI.

Ankle pressure

- Position the cuff around the ankle immediately above the malleoli (protect ulcer if present).
- Locate leg pulses by palpation or with the Doppler probe.
- Repeat as for brachial pressure reading.
- Record the ankle pressure as the highest reading of at least 2 pulses on each leg, such as the dorsalis pedis (felt between the first and second metatarsals) and the posterior tibial (felt behind the medial malleolus) pulse.
- Repeat for other leg (Vowden, 1996).

Points to remember when undertaking Doppler assessment

- Do not use any products other than Doppler conductive gel as they can damage the Doppler.
- If the probe is pressed too hard this can stop blood flow and eradicate the signal.
- After using the Doppler device, remove any gel from the probe and clean the tip with an aqueous solution. Alcohol or other disinfectants can cause damage. Remove any gel from the patients skin (McConnell, 2000).

Doppler readings

- The resting ABPI should be greater than 1.
- An ABPI of less than 0.9 indicated some arterial disease.
- An ABPI of 0.8 or less indicates significant arterial disease and compression therapy should not be applied.

Preparations for the treatment of chronic skin ulcers:

- Metronidazole 0.075% and 0.8% gel (Metrogel®, Metrotop®, Rozex®)
- Silver Sulfadiazine 1% Cream (Flamazine®)

Metronidazole

Mode of action

Metronidazole is effective in treating protozoan and anaerobic gram-negative bacterial infections and greatly reduces the odour which accompanies these wound infections, e.g. in necrotic pressure sores. Although its mechanism of action is not fully understood, it is thought to prevent DNA replication and so is bactericidal.

Adverse effects

Local skin irritation.

Nursing Points

The wound should be cleaned and the preparation applied 1–2 times daily. The gel should be applied liberally to flat wounds, and smeared on paraffin gauze and packed loosely into cavity wounds.

Silver sulfadiazine cream (Flamazine®)

This preparation is a sulphonamide. The sulphonamides have a similar function to antibiotics but are developed from chemicals, as opposed to fungi or moulds. Silver sulphadiazine has an antibacterial effect (against gram-negative and gram-positive organisms), and is also effective against yeasts and fungi. It can be applied to leg ulcers and pressure sores.

Mode of action

Bacteria require folic acid if they are to grow. This is produced by an enzymatic reaction within the bacterial cell. The sulphonamides interfere with this reaction and the formation of folic acid is prevented. The bacteria are therefore unable to survive (Henry, 2001).

Contraindications

This preparation should not be given during pregnancy or breastfeeding. It is not recommended for neonates.

Adverse effects

Allergic reaction including stinging and rash.

Nursing Points

This preparation should be applied daily or every 48 h and used with an absorbent, retaining dressing. Silver sulfadiazine should not be used in wounds with high levels of exudate.

Atopic dermatitis

Dermatitis or eczema is an inflammatory disorder of the skin. Individuals who suffer from atopic dermatitis generally have a family history of hypersensitivity reactions. This condition is seen more frequently in children but can persist throughout life (LeMone and Burke, 1996). In adults, areas of the skin become red, thickened, and hardened, and may become infected as a result of scratching.

Evidence supporting the avoidance of house dust mites, wet wraps or other forms of bandaging, and changes in diet, is limited (Charman, 2000). Preparations used to treat atopic eczema involve the use of emollients with topical corticosteroids. Corticosteroids in combination with antimicrobials can be used to treat small, localised areas of infected eczema. Infection can also be treated with antibiotics.

Emollients

Emollients soothe, smooth and hydrate the skin and are used in the treatment of dry skin. The effects of emollient preparations are short lived, and they need to be applied frequently even after improvement occurs. Emollient preparations are available in a variety of presentations. Each of these preparations varies with regard to the water and oil content of the mixture. Preparations with a high water content produce a greater cooling effect on the skin, and so are very effective for individuals suffering from pruritus. Individuals with very severe dry skin may benefit from an emollient with higher oil content. The high oil content produces a greater sealing effect on the skin, and thus prevents water evaporation to a greater extent.

Mode of action

- *Creams* – Creams are oil-in-water emulsions. Their action takes place in two stages (Nathan, 1997). Firstly, following the initial application of the preparation, water is lost from the mixture by both evaporation, and absorption into the skin. This water evaporation has the effect of cooling the skin and alleviating pruritus. Secondly, the water loss from the mixture, combined with the mechanical stress of applying the preparation, causes the emulsion to crack. This cracking releases the oil phase. During this phase, oil is released onto the surface of the skin, sealing it, and preventing any further water evaporating from the skin's surface.

  Creams are generally well absorbed into the skin, are less greasy than ointments, and easier to apply. They therefore tend to be more cosmetically acceptable. Creams are a popular method for the treatment of minor dry skin conditions. Aqueous Cream, is an example of a cream preparation.

- *Ointments* – Ointments are greasy preparations, that do not normally contain water, and are insoluble in water. They are more occlusive than creams. Ointments are particularly effective in chronic, dry lesions. Commonly used ointment bases consist of soft paraffin or a combination of soft, liquid, and hard paraffin. Emulsifying Ointment is an example of this type of preparation.

A wide range of emollient preparations are currently available. However, there is little published evidence of the relative effectiveness of these products, and choice is often a matter of personal preference. All emollient products can be bought over-the-counter. However, some of these products may be very expensive, and are usually supplied on prescription.

Contraindications

Generally, emollients are very safe to use, the only contraindication being sensitivity to the constituents in the preparation. This effect is most notable with hydrous wool fat (lanolin) and should be suspected if an eczematous reaction occurs. Constituents in Aqueous Cream and Emulsifying Ointment include paraffins.

Nursing Points

The administration of an emollient will depend on the condition of the patient. It may be necessary for an individual to have a daily bath containing an emollient, and then to apply further emollients. In other instances, individuals may only require the infrequent application of cream to an area of dry skin.

Individuals with atopic eczema or severe dry skin will benefit from having a bath prior to using an emollient. The bath water will hydrate the skin and therefore provide an extremely good base for the application of these preparations. The bath water must only be lukewarm (approximately 37°C). This is very important, as if it is any hotter, blood vessels will become dilated and any itching may become worse. Emulsifying Ointment can also be used as a bath additive. Approximately 30 g of this mixture should be mixed with hot water and poured into the bath. Following bathing, the skin should be gently patted dry. If an emollient preparation is to be applied to the skin, it should be done so before the skin dries out, and immediately following the bath. Emollients can be applied as often as they are required throughout the day.

Preparations used in the treatment of atopic dermatitis – Topical corticosteroids and antimicrobials:

Topical corticosteroids:

- Alclometasone dipropionate 0.05% cream and ointment (Modrasone®).
- Beclometasone diproprionate 0.025% cream and ointment (Propaderm®).
- Betamethasone 0.01% as valerate in water miscible basis containing coconut oil derivative scalp application (Betacap®).
- Betamethasone 0.01% as valerate in water miscible basis scalp application (Betnovate®).
- Betamethasone 0.05% as diproprionate cream, lotion, and ointment (Diprosone®).
- Betamethasone valerate cream, lotion, and ointment 0.1% as valerate, cream, and ointment at 1 in 4 dilution: betamethasone as 0.025% as valerate (Betnovate® and Betnovate RD®).
- Betamethasone 0.01% as valerate foam scalp application (Bettamousse®).
- Hydrocortisone 1%, urea 10% and lactic acid 5% cream (Calmurid HC®).

- Clobetasone butyrate 0.05% cream and ointment (Eumovate®).
- Desoximetasone 0.05% Oily cream (Stiedex®).
- Fludroxycortide 0.0125% cream and ointment (Haelan®).
- Fluocinolone acetonide cream, gel, and ointment 0.025%, and cream and ointment at 1 in 4 dilution: fluocinolone acetonide 0.00625%, and Cream at 1 in 10 dilution: fluocinolone acetonide 0.0025% (Synalar®, Synalar 1 in 4 Dilution®).
- Fluocinonide 0.05% cream and ointment (Metosyn®).
- Fluocortolone hexanoate 0.25% and fluocortolone pivalate 0.25% cream and ointment (Ultralanumplain®).
- Fluticasone Propionate cream 0.05% and ointment 0.005% (Cutivate®).
- Hydrocortisone 1% and Urea 10% cream (Alphaderm®).
- Hydrocortisone Butyrate 0.1% in aqueous isopropyl alcoholic basis scalp lotion (Locoid®).
- Hydrocortisone 0.25% and crotamiton 10% Cream (Eurax-Hydrocortisone®, Eurax Hc®).
- Hydrocortisone butyrate 0.1% cream, lotion, and ointment (Locoid®).
- Hydrocortisone 0.5% and 1% cream and ointment (Non-proprietary).
- Momtasone furoate 0.1% cream and ointment (Elocon®).
- Momtasone furoate 0.1% in aqueous isopropyl alcoholic basis scalp lotion (Elocon®).

Topical corticosteroids with antimicrobials:

- Clotrimazole 1% and betamethasone 0.05% as dipropionate cream (Lotriderm®).
- Clotrimazole 1% and hydrocortisone 1% cream (Canesten HC®).
- Betamethasone 0.1% as valerate and fusidic acid 3% cream (Fusibet®).
- Betamethasone 0.1% as valerate and clioquinol 3% cream and ointments (Betnovate-C®).
- Hydrocortisone butyrate 0.1% and chlorquinaldol 3% cream and ointment (Locoid C®).
- Hydrocortisone acetate 1% and fusidic acid 2% cream and ointment (Fucidin H®).
- Hydrocortisone 1% and potassium hydroxyquinoline sulphate 0.5% cream (Quinocort®).
- Hydrocortisone 1% and oxytetracycline hydrochloride 3% (Terra-Cortril Ointment®).
- Triamcinolone acetonide 0.1% and chlortetracycline hydrochloride 3% ointment (Aurecort®).
- Clobetasone butyrate 0.05%, oxytetracycline 3% as calcium salt and nystatin 100,000 units/g (Trimovate Cream®).

- Miconazole nitrate 2% and hydrocortisone 1% cream and ointment (Daktacort®).
- Nystatin cream 100,000 units/g, hydrocortisone 0.5%, and chlorhexidine hydrochloride 1%, ointment nystatin 100,000 units/g, hydrocortisone 0.5% and chlorhexidine acetate 1% (Nystaform-HC®).
- Hydrocortisone 0.5%, nystatin 100,000 units/g, benzalkonium chloride solution 0.2%, dimeticone '350' 10% cream (Timodine®).

Topical corticosteroid with antibacterial:

- Fluocinolone Acetonide 0.025% and cleoquinol 3% cream and ointment (Synalar C®).

Nursing Points

The treatment of atopic dermatitis includes the regular use of emollients, topical corticosteroids for acute episodes and oral antibiotics for exacerbation of infection (MCA, 2001). These must be prescribed by a doctor for this condition. The topical corticosteroid applied should be the least potent preparation that is effective (*see* page 109/110). In mild to moderate atopic eczema it should be used for periods of 1–2 weeks in conjunction with an emollient. A more potent corticosteroid may be required in more severe cases followed by a weaker preparation. An emollient should also be applied (BNF, 2002).

For mode of action, contraindications, adverse effects, and nursing points, see under skin candidiasis for corticosteroids and compound preparations. For oral antibiotics, *see* Chapter 2.

Contact dermatitis

Contact dermatitis is a localised inflammatory reaction which can be caused by chemical irritation or, hypersensitivity to an allergen. Treatment involves identification and avoidance of the allergen or irritant, emollients, and topical corticosteroids in acute episodes (MCA, 2001) (*See* atopic dermatitis).

Seborrhoeic dermatitis

Seborrhoeic dermatitis is an inflammatory disorder involving the scalp, eyebrows, eyelids, ear canals, nasolabial folds, axillae, and trunk. It can be seen in all age groups and is associated with an overgrowth of the commensal yeast *Pityrosporum* (MCA, 2001).

In the infants it is known as 'cradle cap' (LeMone and Burke, 1996). Lesions are orange and scaly, crusted and greasy.

Preparations used in the treatment of seborrhoeic dermatitis:

- Topical antifungals – see skin candidiasis
- Corticosteroid gels and lotions – see atopic dermatitis

Aston *et al.*, 1998). Head lice may be treated by three methods: mechanical clearance using the wet combing method; by using an insecticide preparation; or by other treatments involving alternative remedies such as tea-tree oil and other herbal substances. While there is some evidence that insecticides are effective, there is still no published evidence that mechanical methods such as 'Bug Busting' or alternative remedies are effective.

A diagnosis of head louse infection cannot be made with certainty unless a living, moving louse is found. Use of a louse comb is more efficient and much quicker than direct visual examination (Mumcuoglu *et al.*, 2001), and according to Aston *et al.* (1998) the only reliable method of diagnosing current, active infection is by detection combing. The wet combing method is the best method of detecting live lice. This involves washing the hair in the normal manner, using an ordinary shampoo. An ordinary conditioner can then be applied to the hair. It is then combed with a fine tooth detector comb whilst still wet. The hair should be combed in good lighting over a white cloth or paper towel in order to see the lice as they are removed. This process should take about 15 min.

Treatment with insecticides

According to Aston *et al.* (1998) the cardinal rule before beginning treatment with insecticides, is that this treatment method should not be used unless a living, moving louse has been found on the head of at least one family member. Detection combing of all members should be undertaken, and only those found to be infected should be treated.

Malathion, carbaryl, and the pyrethroids are all effective against head lice. In some health authorities, headlice are managed according to a local policy that rotates the use of these insecticides over a 2 or 3 year period. This attempts to reduce the risk of lice developing resistance to the preparations. These procedures of rotating insecticides are however, becoming less popular. Nurses with prescriber status should follow local policy guidelines when making prescribing decisions. Current UK practice involves individual management of each proven case using a mosaic of treatments (National Prescribing Centre, 1999). This is explained in Figure 6.3. This attempts to help overcome the development of resistance.

All three of these insecticidal groups are more effective as lotions rather than shampoos. In addition, the alcohol-based lotions are more effective than the aqueous lotions.

Contraindications

Malathion, carbaryl, and the pyrethroids should not be applied to broken skin or secondarily infected skin. When used, care should be taken to avoid the eyes with all preparations.

Alcoholic lotions should be avoided in patients with asthma and in small children.

All children under 6 months should be treated under the care of a physician.

Permethrin should be avoided in pregnancy and if breastfeeding.

Figure 6.3 – An example of a mosaic approach to the treatment of head lice

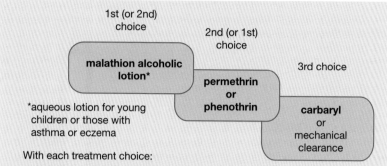

1st (or 2nd) choice

malathion alcoholic lotion*

2nd (or 1st) choice

permethrin or phenothrin

3rd choice

carbaryl or mechanical clearance

*aqueous lotion for young children or those with asthma or eczema

With each treatment choice:

- Use two applications of insecticide, seven days apart.
- 2–3 days after final application of insecticide: check hair thoroughly with a plastic detector comb.
- If adult lice are present then go on to next choice of treatment. Always thoroughly investigate the reason for treatment failure.

(Modified from the National Prescribing Centre, 1999)

Adverse effects

Malathion, carbaryl, and the pyrethroids may all cause skin irritation. In addition, permethrin may cause erythema, stinging, rashes, and oedema.

Nursing Points

Insecticides should not be used as prophylaxis for head lice. The wet combing method, however, may be used as a preventive measure.

When prescribing a preparation, always observe the contraindications and precautions. Factors to consider are: age of the patient, whether pregnant or breast feeding, the presence of other skin problems, and whether suffering from asthma.

Manufacturer's instructions must be followed for the specific preparation prescribed. A contact time of 12 h is recommended for most lotions and liquids. The parent or patient will need instruction on where and how it should be applied, and the length of time it must remain on the body to have its maximum effect.

A course of treatment for head lice is usually two applications of a preparation, 1 week apart. The second application aims to kill any remaining lice hatching from eggs that may have survived the first application.

Chlorine inactivates malathion, so patients should be advised to avoid swimming pools within 1 week of treatment.

Close contacts of those infested should be followed up and if necessary should be treated.

Further treatment with a different preparation will be required for those who remain symptomatic. Evidence of a secondary infection will necessitate a referral to the patient's General Practitioner (GP) for possible antibiotic therapy.

Li Wan Po (1990) suggests that in order for nurses to avoid excessive exposure to insecticides, gloves should be worn by those nurses involved in the application of these preparations.

Mechanical clearance

This whole method of treatment needs to be repeated every 3–4 days over a period of 2 weeks (Cook, 1998). The presence of conditioner on the hair is thought to make the hair slippery and easier to detach the lice from the hair shaft. 'Bug Buster Kits' are available from the charity, Community Hygiene Concern, which promotes the wetcombing method. The 1998 Kit (with an improved comb) is now undergoing independent evaluation in comparison with licensed products (Ibarra, 2001).

Management of pubic lice

Malathion, phenothrin, and permethrin will treat pubic lice effectively.

Contraindications and adverse effects

See previous section on the management of head lice.

Nursing Points

Alcoholic preparations are not recommended due to irritation of excoriated skin and genitalia. Aqueous preparations should be applied to all parts of the body and not just the axillae and groins. The preparation should remain on the body for 12 h or overnight. As for the treatment of head lice, a second application is necessary after 1 week.

Management of body lice

These lice only visit the skin for a supply of fresh blood, therefore clothes will be the main source of lice. All clothing and bedding of infested patients should be treated. After washing the clothes and bedding, use of a hot air tumble dryer will ensure destruction of lice and eggs remaining in the material.

Insecticides may be necessary, however, advice from a physician should be sought.

Scabies

Sarcoptes scabiei is the mite responsible for scabies, which has its highest incidence in teenagers, and children aged 8–12 years (Nathan, 1997). Scabies infestation is also increasing, with outbreaks in closed communities such as hospitals and nursing homes (Li Wan Po, 1990). Personal contact is normally necessary to acquire the mite, with clothing and bedding not thought to be important in the transmission of infection.

The female mite burrows through the stratum corneum of the skin and lays its eggs just above the boundary between the epidermis and dermis (see Figure 6.1). The mite normally remains there for the duration of its life, which is approximately 30 days. Two or three eggs are laid daily, which hatch after about 4 days. Common sites for burrows are the finger webs and wrists. However, the palms of the hands, soles of the feet, penis, scrotum, buttocks, and axillae may be involved.

An allergic response to the mite's coat, saliva, and faeces is thought to be responsible for the major symptom of severe itching. Areas of itching may be widespread, with secondary skin infection and skin damage present, due to excessive scratching. Secondary infection may take the form of impetigo or pustules.

The presence of burrows aids confirmation of diagnosis, and these can be scraped to reveal the mite and eggs (Mead, 1996).

Preparations for the treatment of scabies:

- Malathion alcoholic lotions (Prioderm® lotion)
- Malathion aqueous lotions (Derbac-M® liquid, Quellada M® liquid)
- Permethrin dermal cream (Lyclear® dermal cream)

Contraindications and adverse effects

See previous section on the management of head lice.

Nursing Points

As alcoholic preparations are more likely to cause irritation to excoriated skin and the genitalia, aqueous preparations are preferable.

They should be applied to clean, dry, and cool skin, covering all body surfaces. A hot bath is not necessary and this may, indeed, increase systemic absorption and remove the drugs from their site of action. Particular attention should be paid to the finger webs and brushing lotion under the ends of the nails. The scalp, neck, face, and ears do need to be treated in the very young and the elderly. These areas should also be treated in the immunocompromised and those that are experiencing treatment failure.

Patients should not wash their hands after application, as hands need to be treated. Reapplication is essential after handwashing.

All members of an affected household should be treated.

Provided the preparation has been applied adequately, then one application is usually sufficient.

Once only, normal laundering is sufficient for the patient's clothing and bedding.

It is normal for itching to persist for 2–3 weeks after treatment, so itching should not be regarded as treatment failure. Calamine lotion or crotamiton cream may be applied to try and control itching. Itching that persists after 3 weeks may mean treatment failure and a referral to the GP should be made to confirm the diagnosis.

Evidence of a secondary infection also warrants a GP referral as antibiotic therapy may be required.

Urticaria

Urticaria is an allergic skin condition commonly called 'nettle rash' or 'hives'. The area of skin affected becomes intensely itchy. There are localised areas of oedema with surrounding erythema. The cause of this condition is frequently not found, although it can be triggered by hot or cold temperatures or an allergy (MCA, 2001). Oral antihistamines are effective in this condition. If urticaria is chronic or reoccurring a medical assessment is necessary.

Preparations for the treatment of urticaria:

- Acrivastine capsules 8 mg capsules (Semprex®, Benadryl Allergy Relief®)
- Alimemazine tartrate syrup 7.5 mg/5 ml (Vellergan®)
- Alimemazine tartrate tablets 10 mg (Vellergan®)
- Azelastine hydrochloride aqueous nasal spray 140 µg per spray (Rhinolast®)
- Cetirizine hydrochloride oral solution 5 mg/5 ml (Zirtek®)
- Cetirizine hydrochloride tablets 10 mg (Zirtek®)
- Fexofenadine hydrochloride tablets 120 mg (Telfast® 120)
- Levocabastine 0.05% hydrochloride aqueous nasal spray (Levostin®)
- Loratadine syrup 5 mg/5 ml (Clarityn®)
- Loratadine tablets 10 mg (Clarityn®)

See allergic rhinitis (Chapter 5) for the mode of action, contraindications, adverse effects, and nursing points for these products.

References

Alexander J (1984). *Arthropods and Human Skin*. Berlin: Springer-Verlag.
Aston R, Duggal H, Simpson J (1998). *Head lice. Report for Consultants in Communicable Disease Control (CCDCs)*. The Public Health Medicine Environmental Group Executive Committee.
BNF (2002). London: British Medical Association and the Royal Pharmaceutical Society of Great Britain.

Burgess I (2000). Head lice. *Clinical Evidence* 4: 975–978.

Bux M (1996). Selection and use of wound dressings. *Wound Care for Pharmacists*. Summer issue: 11–16.

Charman C (2000). Atopic eczema. *Clinical Evidence* 4: 944–956.

Cook R (1998). Treatment of head lice. *Nursing Standard* 12(18): 49–52.

Cullum N, Nelson E, Nixon J (2000). Pressure sores. *Clinical Evidence* 4: 1159–1166.

Dealey C. (1994). *The Care of Wounds*. Oxford: Blackwell Scientific Publications.

DoH (1996). *The Prevention and Treatment of Head Lice*. (Leaflet, March 1996 (07)). London: DoH.

DTB (1996). Augmentin reconsidered. *Drug and Therapeutic Bulletin* 34: 76–78.

Dunford C (1997). Management of recurrent pilonidal sinus. *Nursing Times* 93(32): 64.

Fentem PH (1986). Elastic hosiery. *Pharmacy Update* 5: 200–205.

Fletcher A, Cullum N, Sheldon TA (1997). A systematic review of compression treatment for venous leg ulcers. *British Medical Journal* 315: 576–580.

Galbraith A, Bullock S, Manias E, Hunt B, Richards A (1999). *Fundamentals of Pharmacology*. UK: Addison Wesley Longman Ltd.

Graham-Brown R, Burns T (1990). *Lecture notes on dermatology* (6th edn). Oxford: Blackwell Scientific Publications.

Henry JA (2001). *The British Medical Association Concise Guide to Medicines and Drugs*. London: Dorling Kindersley.

Hopkins SJ (1999). *Drugs and Pharmacology for Nurses*. Edinburgh: Churchill Livingstone.

Ibarra J (2001). Head lice: changing the costly chemotherapy culture. *British Journal of Community Nursing* 6(3): 146–151.

LeMone P, Burke K (1996). *Medical Surgical Nursing*. California: Addison-Wesley.

Li Wan Po A (1990). Non-Prescription Drugs (2nd edn). Oxford: Blackwell Scientific Publications.

Maibach HI (1974). Percutaneous penetration of some pesticides and herbicides in man. *Toxicology and Applied Pharmacology* 28: 126–132.

Martini FH (2000). *Fundamentals of Anatomy and Physiology* (5th edn). New Jersey: Prentice Hall International.

Maunder JW (1977). Parasites and man. Human lice: Biology and control. *Royal Society of Health Journal* 1: 29–32.

Maunder JW (1983). The appreciation of lice. Proceedings of the Royal Institute of Great Britain. 55: 1–31.

MCA (2001). *Extended Prescribing of Prescription Only Medicines By Independent Nurse Prescribers*. London: MCA.

McConnell EA (2000). Using a Doppler device (do's and don'ts). *Nursing 2000*. July, 17.

Mead M (1996). Scabies and lice. *Practice Nurse* 20 Sept: 336–337.

Mumcuoglu KY, Friger M, Ioffe-Uspensky I, Ben-Ishaii F, Miller J (2001). Louse comb versus direct visual examination for the diagnosis of head louse infestations. *Pediatric Dermatology* 18(1): 9–12.

Nathan A (1997). Products for skin problems. *The Pharmaceutical Journal* 259: 606–610.

Nathan A (1997). Treatments for scabies. *The Pharmaceutical Journal* 259: 331–332.

National Prescribing Centre (1999). Management of head louse infection. *Prescribing Nurse Bulletin* 1(4): 13–16.

Nelson E, Cullum N, Jones J (2000). Venous leg ulcers. *Clinical Evidence* 4: 1167–1177.

Sadler C (1997). A lousy headache. *Community Nurse* 3(10): 8.

Scowen P (1995). Government restricts the use of carbaryl for head lice. *Professional Care of Mother and Child* 5(6): 163–165.

Thomas S (1990). *Wound Management and Dressings*. London: The Pharmaceutical Press.

Vowden KR (1996). Hand-held Doppler assessment for peripheral arterial disease. *Journal of Wound Care* 5(3): 125–128.

Winter GD (1962). Formation of the scab and the rate of epithelialisation of superficial wounds in the skin of the young domestic pig. *Nature* 193: 293–294.

Worrall G (2000). Herpes labialis. *Clinical Evidence* 4: 979–984.

Chapter 7

Preparations for Minor Injuries of the Musculoskeletal System

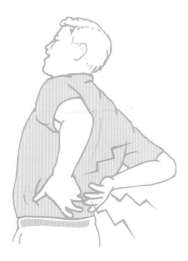

This chapter will provide the nurse prescriber with the relevant anatomy and physiology underpinning minor injuries affecting the musculoskeletal system together with the recommended management and treatment.

Skeletal Muscles

Skeletal muscles (also called striped or striated muscles) are attached by tendons to the bones of the skeleton. There are over 600 of these muscles and they are arranged in the body in parallel bundles, the cells forming a striped pattern. Skeletal muscles are voluntary, i.e. we are able to control their action. They move a part of the body by contracting and pulling on the bone to which they are attached.

Skeletal muscles are arranged and work in pairs, i.e. one on either side of a bone. This enables the bone to be moved in either direction. They also work in groups adjusting for each of the activities that the body makes. For example, when changing our position, certain muscles are forced to take up the strain of the new position, and become contracted, others are able to relax as the strain is taken away.

Bones and Joints

Bones and joints make up the framework of the body. Their flexibility enables them to adapt to the demands placed upon them throughout life. Exercise plays an important role in maintaining the strength of bones and the suppleness of joints.

Bones

Bones have a number of functions including:

- providing the skeletal framework and protecting the organs of the body
- enabling movement
- storage of mineral salts

Bones are slightly soft and flexible, as over 30% of each bone is made up of water. They require nutrients and detect sensation and therefore, have their own blood and nerve supply. The hard, dense, outer shell of a bone is called compact bone. This is made up of tiny cylindrical units known as Haversian systems, which provide much of the strength of bone. The tube-shaped Haversian units lie in the direction of the greatest stresses on the bone. For example, in the femur they lie lengthways in the bone shaft, so the bone resists buckling. Within the compact bone is a spongy substance known as spongy, trabecular, or cancellous bone, and in the centre of the bone is a soft jelly-like substance called bone marrow.

Joints

Cartilage is found at the end of bones where they come into contact. Bones are linked to each other by ligaments to form a joint. Joints can be fibrous, cartilaginous or, synovial. The bones of the skull are held together tightly by fibrous tissue, i.e. fibrous joints. Cartilaginous joints such as vertebral joints allow greater flexibility, and synovial joints enable a further range of movement.

Lever systems and movement

Movement in human beings occurs as a result of lever systems. A lever can be visualised as a rigid bar that rotates around a pivot or fulcrum. A lever moves a load using effort. There are three main types of lever systems within the body. In each system the bone is the lever, the muscles supplying the effort, and the load is the body parts, supported by the bone.

The neck joint is the first-order lever (Figure 7.1). In this type of lever, the fulcrum is positioned between the load and the effort. In the second-order lever system (Figure 7.2), the load is placed between the fulcrum and the effort, e.g. when standing on tiptoe. In third-order levers (Figure 7.3), the effort is in the middle between the fulcrum and the load, e.g. the elbow joint.

Muscles of the Neck and Vertebral Column

Muscles originating from the head, neck, and trunk move the head. The deep back muscles arising from the vertebral column effect movement of the trunk of the body. These muscles and muscles of the trunk also have a role in maintaining body posture and the normal curvature of the spine. Superficial back muscles control the movements of the upper limbs and shoulder girdle (Marieb, 2000).

Extending from the sacrum to the skull is a column of deep muscles. This column is made up of a number of muscles of different length. When individual muscles are pulled, vertebrae are caused to extend or rotate on lower vertebrae. In this way,

Figure 7.1 – First-order lever

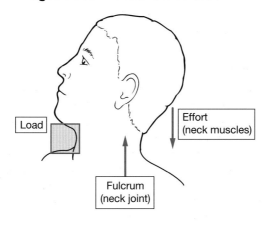

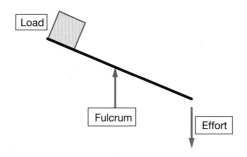

the vertebral column is able to move smoothly. Shorter muscles which extend between vertebrae help to stabilise the spine.

Acute, uncomplicated low back pain

Acute low back pain involves the lumbar, lumbarsacral, or sacroiliac areas of the back. It is most frequently due to strains in the muscle or tendons caused by overuse or abnormal stress. It affects both men and women and is prevalent in individuals aged between their late twenties and mid fifties (LeMone and Burke, 1996).

Preparations for the treatment of acute, uncomplicated low back pain:

- Ibuprofen granules 600 mg/sachet and syrup 100 mg/5 ml (Brufen®)
- Ibuprofen modified release tablets and capsules 800 mg (Brufen Retard®)
- Ibuprofen tablets 200 mg, 400 mg, 600 mg, 800 mg, and suspension 100 mg/1 ml (Brufen®)

- Aspirin 300 mg tablets, enteric coated tablets, dispersable tablets, and suppositories
- Codeine phosphate 15 mg, 30 mg, and 60 mg tablets
- Dihydrocodeine 60 mg in modified release tablets (DHC Continus®)
- Dihydrocodeine 40 mg tablets (DF118 Forte®)
- Dihydrocodeine 30 mg tablets
- Nefopam hydrochloride 30 mg tablets (Acupan®)
- Paracetamol preparations 120–500 mg per dose

For mode of action, contraindications, adverse effects, and nursing points for these preparations, *see* Chapter 3. Further nursing points are outlined below.

Figure 7.2 – Second-order lever

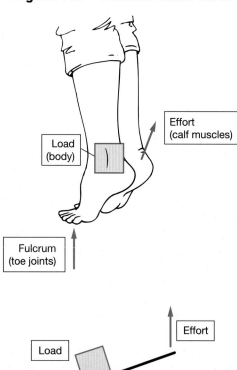

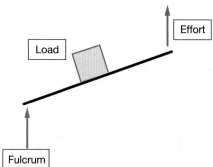

Figure 7.3 – Third-order lever

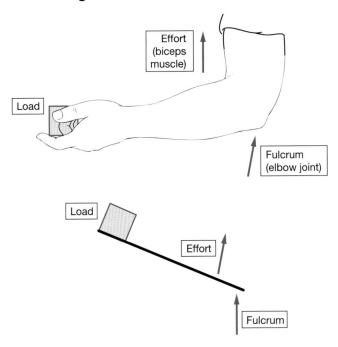

Nursing Points

The patient's age, description of the symptoms and their duration, the impact of the symptoms on the activity of the patient, the response of the patient to any previous therapy, and any psychological and socio-economic problems are important areas in the assessment of the patient complaining of acute, uncomplicated low back pain (Waddell *et al.*, 1999).

Nerve root pain or any possible, serious spinal pathology must be identified during the initial assessment. Acute, uncomplicated, low back pain generally presents between the ages of 20 and 55 years, is experienced in the lumbosacral region, buttocks and thighs. The pain is mechanical in nature and varies with physical activity and time. The patient is generally well and the prognosis is good, 90% of patients recovering from an acute attack within 6 weeks (Waddell *et al.*, 1999).

If the patient complains of unilateral leg pain (worse than the low back pain), radiating to the foot or toes and accompanied by numbness and paraesthesia, reduced straight leg raising, and motor, sensory or reflex changes, these are symptoms of nerve root pain. The patient must be referred for a medical assessment. Fifty percent of individuals with this type of pain recover within 6 weeks (Waddell *et al.*, 1999).

A number of 'red flags' indicating possible serious spinal pathology have been identified by Waddell *et al.* (1999). These 'red flags' include symptoms and signs of cauda equina syndrome (difficulty with micturition, loss of anal sphincter tone or faecal incontinence, and saddle anaesthesia about the anus, perineum or genitalia), widespread neurological involvement and severe or progressive motor weakness.

Other 'red flags' include:

- Violent trauma, e.g. a fall from a height, road traffic accident.
- If the individual is under the age of 20 or, if the symptoms present over 55.
- Constant, progressive and non-mechanical pain.
- Thoracic pain.
- Past medical history of carcinoma.
- If the patient has been taking systemic steroids.
- Drug abuse, HIV.
- If the individual is systemically unwell.
- If there is weight loss.
- Persisting, severe restriction of lumbar flexion.
- Structural deformity (Waddell et al., 1999).

A person suffering from acute uncomplicated low back pain should be encouraged to stay active, advised to maintain the correct posture and to take care when lifting or bending (Waddell et al., 1999). Paracetamol should be the first treatment of choice. Ibuprofen is recommended if Paracetamol is ineffective (CSM, 1994). If symptoms are severe, and muscle relaxants or strong opioids are necessary, a medical assessment is required (for further guidance on the management of acute and low back pain see the Royal College of General Practitioners – Waddell et al., 1999).

Acute, uncomplicated neck pain

Acute neck pain is usually due to a sprain or, by a persistent or permanent twisting of the neck causing an abnormality in the position of the head (torticollis). Whiplash injury to the neck and muscle spasm might cause this condition. Treatment and management involves the continuation of normal activity and drug management as for acute, uncomplicated, low back pain. As in acute, uncomplicated, low back pain, medical assessment is necessary if there is any nerve root pain or other neurological symptoms, if muscle relaxants or opioids are required, or if the 'red flags' indicating a possible serious spinal pathology are present.

Soft Tissue Injury

Common soft tissue injuries include contusions, sprains and strains.

Contusions

A contusion involves bleeding into the soft tissue due to the rupture of a small blood vessel resulting from a blunt force, e.g. a punch. A haematoma is a contusion with a large amount of bleeding. Over time the blood is reabsorbed.

Table 7.1 – Sprains and strains

Sprain	Strain
• Injury to a ligament resulting from a twisting motion • Possible joint instability • Pain, oedema and swelling • Pain on joint movement	• Microscopic tear in the muscle • Dull or sharp pain • Isometric contraction of the muscle increases pain • Swelling and local tenderness (LeMone and Burke, 1996)

Sprains

When a ligament is overstretched or torn, i.e. as a result of a twisting motion, a sprain results. This is also accompanied by bleeding into the soft tissue. Sprains commonly occur in the ankle as a result of external rotation. In this instance, the ankle moves in the opposite direction to the body.

Strains

A strain is a small tear in the muscle accompanied by bleeding into the tissue. A muscle becomes strained if overextended, e.g. if lifting a heavy object. Table 7.1 compares sprains and strains.

Preparations for the treatment of soft tissue injury:

- Ibuprofen granules 600 mg/sachet and syrup 100 mg/5 ml (Brufen®)
- Ibuprofen modified release tablets and capsules 800 mg (Brufen Retard®)
- Ibuprofen tablets 200 mg, 400 mg, 600 mg, 800 mg, and suspension 100 mg/1ml (Brufen®)
- Piroxicam 0.5% (Feldene® Gel)
- Ibuprofen 10% (Fenbid® Forte Gel)
- Ibuprofen 10% (Ibugel® Forte Gel)
- Ketoprofen 2.5% (Oruvail® Gel)
- Ketoprofen 2.5% (Powergel®)
- Felbinac Foam 3.17%, Felbinac Gel 3% (Traxam® Foam and Gel)
- Diclofenac diethylammonium salt 1.16% (Voltarol Emugel®)
- Aspirin 300 mg tablets, enteric coated tablets, dispersable tablets and suppositories
- Codeine phosphate 15 mg, 30 mg, and 60 mg tablets
- Dihydrocodeine 60 mg in modified release tablets (DHC Continus®)
- Dihydrocodeine 40 mg tablets (DF118 Forte®)
- Dihydrocodeine 30 mg tablets

- Nefopam hydrochloride 30 mg tablets (Acupan®)
- Paracetamol preparations 120–500 mg per dose

For mode of action, contraindications, adverse effects and nursing points for pain relief and NSAIDs, see Chapter 3. Further nursing points for the management of sprains and strains are outlined below.

Nursing Points

The strain or sprain may benefit from ice, compression, and elevation, following the injury (MCA, 2001). However, this will depend on its severity. Normal physical activity should be resumed as soon as possible and compression discontinued. The application of local heat, and topical NSAIDs can be effective. Topical NSAIDs, in large quantities, may result in systemic effects (for a discussion of NSAIDs see Chapter 3). These preparations should not be used with an occlusive dressing and the patient should be cautioned against exposing the treated area to excessive sunlight in order to avoid photosensitivity.

Skeletal muscle spasm in palliative care

Painful muscle spasm or cramp may last from a few seconds to many hours or days. In palliative care, patients may develop cramp due to one of several causes. Twycross (1997) identifies some of the causes of cramps. Cramp may arise in a muscle close to a painful bone metastasis; it may be drug-induced; other causes include meningeal metastases, nerve compression, peripheral neuropathy, polymyositis, and concurrent spinal degeneration.

It is beyond the scope of this book to consider the detailed management of problems in palliative care. However, products are available in the extended formulary for the treatment of skeletal muscle spasm in this patient group. Appropriately trained nurses may prescribe the following products, having considered treating reversible causes and the use of physical therapies such as massage and relaxation techniques.

Preparations for the treatment of skeletal muscle spasm in palliative care:

- Baclofen tablets (Lioresal®)
- Dantrolene capsules (Dantrium®)
- Diazepam tablets and injection

Mode of action

Baclofen acts by stimulating GABA receptors in the spinal cord. As a consequence of this, the reflex muscle contractions associated with some forms of muscle spasm are suppressed. In addition there is an analgesic effect, as the release of substance P (a spinal chemical mediator of pain transmission) is blocked (Galbraith et al., 1999).

Dantrolene acts directly on the skeletal muscle fibres, and inhibits the release of calcium from the sarcoplasmic reticulum of the muscle cell. It reduces the excitation-contraction coupling process, but does not abolish contraction of skeletal muscle (Waller and Renwick, 1994). Diazepam, like baclofen, also stimulates GABA receptors. The mode of action, contraindications, and adverse effects of diazepam have been discussed previously in Chapter 3.

Contraindications

Baclofen is contraindicated in peptic ulceration. Caution should be taken in psychiatric disorders, cerebrovascular disease, renal, respiratory and hepatic impairment, epilepsy and hypertonic bladder.

Dantrolene is contraindicated in acute muscle spasm and hepatic impairment.

Adverse effects

Baclofen frequently produces nausea, drowsiness, and sedation. Less common problems include dizziness, confusion, ataxia, headache, hallucinations, euphoria, insomnia, depression, tremor, nystagmus, paraesthesias, convulsions, respiratory depression, cardiac depression, hypotension, dry mouth, urinary, and gastrointestinal disturbance. Some rare adverse effects are altered liver function tests, visual disorders, taste changes, rashes, and increased sweating.

Dantrolene may cause dizziness, fatigue, drowsiness, malaise, headache, convulsions, insomnia, visual disturbance, muscle weakness, nausea, vomiting, constipation, transient diarrhoea, hepatotoxicity, urinary frequency and incontinence, haematuria, crystalluria, and rashes.

Nursing Points

Baclofen should be taken with food to reduce gastrointestinal symptoms. Patients should be informed of potential adverse effects and told to report them. In order to avoid the major adverse effect of sedation, the dose of this preparation should be increased gradually. This drug should not be discontinued abruptly but should be gradually reduced over a period of 1–2 weeks. Drowsiness may affect the patient's ability to undertake other skilled tasks. An enhanced sedative effect occurs if alcohol is consumed and should therefore be avoided. Other CNS depressant drugs should also be avoided.

Dantrolene should be administered with meals, and the dose increased slowly. When discontinued, the dose should be tapered off slowly. The patient should be made aware of the adverse effects and when to report them. As with baclofen, the patient's ability to drive and undertake skilled tasks may be impaired, and alcohol should be avoided. Liver function should be assessed at intervals.

Patients should be made aware of the adverse effects of diazepam. The ability to drive and undertake skilled tasks may be affected. Alcohol should be avoided. The drug should not be stopped abruptly after long-term use.

References

CSM (1994). Current problems in pharmacovigilance. *Committee for Safety of Medicines* 20: 9–11.

Galbraith A, Bullock S, Manias E, Hunt B, Richards A (1999). *Fundamentals of Pharmacology*. UK: Addison Wesley Longman Ltd.

LeMone P, Burke K (1996). *Medical Surgical Nursing*. California: Addison-Wesley.

Marieb EN (2000). *Human Anatomy and Physiology* (5th edn). New York: Benjamin Cummings.

MCA (2001). *Extended Prescribing of Prescription Only Medicines By Independent Nurse Prescribers*. London: MCA.

Twycross R (1997). *Symptom Management in Advanced Cancer* (2nd edn). Abingdon: Radcliffe Medical Press.

Waddell G, McIntosh A, Hutchinson A, Feder G, Lewis M (1999). *Low Back Pain*. Evidence Review. London: Royal College of General Practitioners.

Waller D, Renwick A (1994). *Principles of Medical Pharmacology*. London: Balliere Tindall.

Chapter 8

Products and Preparations Affecting the Reproductive System

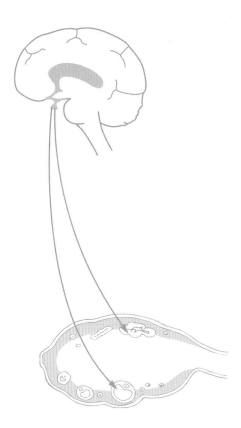

A variety of contraceptive preparations and devices are listed in the extended formulary and available for appropriately trained nurses to prescribe. This chapter commences with an overview of the female reproductive system, sperm transport and fertilisation. The mechanisms by which the diaphragm and cap (female barrier methods of contraception), and spermicides work are then discussed. The chapter moves on to look at the reproductive cycle and the associated hormones and describes the mode of action of combined oral contraception (COC), the progestogen-only-pill (POP), injectable contraceptives and emergency contraception. Bacterial vaginosis, vulvovaginal candidiasis, dysmenorrhoea, and balanitis are conditions of the reproductive system for which nurses are able to prescribe. These conditions, their treatment and management are examined in the remainder of the chapter.

The Female Reproductive System

The female reproductive system comprises of the following:

- ovaries
- uterus
- uterine tubes
- vagina
- external genitalia

The broad ligament, a double layer of serous membrane or mesentery, encases, supports and stabilises the ovaries, uterine tubes, and uterus (Figure 8.1).

The ovaries

The ovaries or female gonads lie within the peritoneal cavity, one on either side of the pelvis. Each of these structures are secured to the uterus by the mesovarium, the ovarian ligament, and the suspensory ligament. The ovaries produce oestrogens and also contain the ova. Oogenesis or the production of ova, occurs monthly (between puberty and menopause) with one gamete, a secondary oocyte, being released every 28 days.

The uterus

The uterus, a hollow pear shaped organ, is situated behind the urinary bladder. The uterus usually leans forward within the pelvis and the cervix points backwards,

Figure 8.1 – Female reproductive system (longitudinal cross-section)

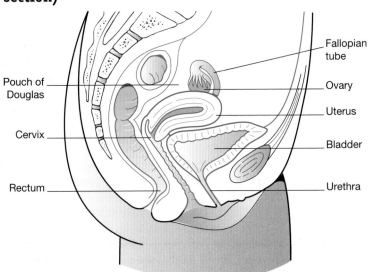

Pouch of Douglas

Cervix

Rectum

Fallopian tube

Ovary

Uterus

Bladder

Urethra

i.e. it is antiverted. The uterus removes waste products, supplies nutrients and protects the developing embryo and foetus (Martini, 2000). It is divided into:

- *The body, or corpus* – This is the larger of the two areas. The fundus (also part of the body) is situated above the junction of the uterine tubes. This structure is comprised primarily of muscle or myometrium and is lined by glandular tissue, i.e. endometrium. The physiological demands of the foetus are supported by the endometrium. This layer changes with the different phases of the uterine cycle, and during menstruation, part of the endometrium is shed.

- *The cervix* – This is the lower region of the uterus that extends into the vagina where it forms a curved surface that surrounds an external opening or the cervical os. The cervical os opens into the cervical canal which, at the internal opening or os, leads into the uterine cavity of the body. The cervix consists of little muscle tissue and is mainly made of connective tissue. The epithelial tissue lining the cervix contains cervical glands. The secretions from these glands vary throughout the menstrual cycle. Suspensory ligaments, a broad ligament, skeletal muscles, and fascia of the pelvic floor, stabilise and support the uterus.

The uterine tubes

The uterine tubes are about 12 cm in length and are positioned between the uterus and ovaries. The infundibulum is the portion of the uterine tube closest to the ovary. The infundibulum is wider in comparison to the rest of the tube and ends in a number of fingerlike projections called fimbriae. Fluid from the peritoneal cavity is pulled into each uterine tube by the movement of these fimbrae. Following ovulation, an oocyte is transported to the uterus. This process is facilitated by contraction of the muscular walls of each uterine tube and the beating of cilia which line each tube. The tube also provides a nutrient rich environment for the spermatozoa and fertilised oocyte.

The vagina

The vagina, is comprised of bundles of smooth muscle. This structure extends between the uterus and the female external genitalia and is parallel to the rectum. The lining of the vagina is kept moist by secretions from the cervical glands. These secretions provide nutrients for resident bacteria and prevent the growth of pathogens. The acidic environment of the vagina can affect the motility of sperm but buffer solutions contained within semen enable successful fertilisation to occur.

The vagina and the urethra pass through the pelvic floor and then through the perineum. A sphincter is formed, around the opening of the vagina, when both the pelvic and perineal muscles contract.

The external genitalia

The vulva contains the female external genitalia. These consist of the labia majora and minora, and the clitoris. Surrounding the vaginal and urethral opening are also sebaceous, sweat and mucus-secreting glands. The mons pubis is situated on the

Figure 8.2 – Female reproductive system (transverse section)

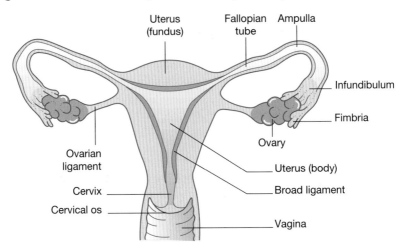

Figure 8.3 – Female external genitalia

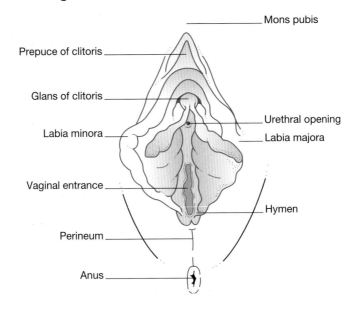

outer limits of the vulva. Adipose tissue under the skin anterior to the pubic symphysis causes this structure to bulge.

During sexual activity, sperm are propelled from the male reproductive tract in two stages – emission and ejaculation. Emission involves the contraction of smooth muscle in the vas deferens, seminal vesicles and prostate gland. This contraction expels secretions into the urethra. Ejaculation, which involves the contraction of striated muscle at the base of the penis, then expels sperm into the woman's vagina.

Sperm transport and fertilisation

Within hours of ejaculation, sperm reach the uterine tubes. Sperm passageway at ovulation is made easier as a result of the cervical mucus becoming thinner. Although it is possible for sperm to survive for up to 7 days in the reproductive tract (Guillebaud, 1997) they usually only survive between 3 and 5 days. During this time they become altered enabling easier adherence to an ovum. Only one sperm normally fertilises the egg and the embryo is then implanted in the endometrial lining.

Female Barrier Methods of Contraception

Both the cap and the diaphragm are barrier methods of contraception, i.e. they prevent fertilisation from occurring by providing a barrier between the egg and sperm.

Diaphragm

The diaphragm (Figure 8.4) is dome shaped and made of latex rubber. It is positioned in the vagina and covers the cervix. If used correctly and in conjunction with a spermicide, it is between 92% and 96% effective (Belfield, 1999). However, if this method is used with a spermicide, but not used carefully, its efficacy is much lower during the first year of use, i.e. between 82% and 90% (Bounds, 1994).

There are three different types of diaphragm.

- *The flat spring diaphragm* – This diaphragm is commonly used in women with a cervix either in the anterior or midplane position. It has a flat spring in its rim. The size of this type of diaphragm ranges from 55–95 mm.

- *Coil spring* – This diaphragm contains a coiled spring in its rim and has greater flexibility than the flat spring diaphragm. Some women find the coil spring more comfortable. This is due to the pressure exerted by the rim of the flat spring being too great or, they have strong vaginal muscles. Women with a shallow symphysis pubis may also find the coil spring diaphragm more comfortable. Sizes available are 55–100 mm.

Figure 8.4 – Diaphragm

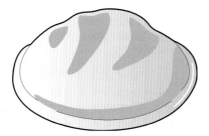

- *Arcing spring diaphragm* – For women who find the flat spring and coil spring difficult to fit, i.e. due to difficulties feeling the cervix or, the posterior position of the cervix, the arcing spring is a useful alternative. Sizes of 65–95 mm are available.

A number of advantages, disadvantages and contraindications for the diaphragm have been described by Everett (1997). These include:

Advantages

- No systemic adverse effects.
- Possible protection against sexually transmitted diseases (not human immunodeficiency virus (HIV)), and cervical cancer.
- Lubrication of the vagina.
- Can be used whilst a woman is menstruating.

Disadvantages

- The rate of effectiveness is low in comparison to other methods of contraception.
- It must be used with care.
- Insertion of the diaphragm and use of spermicides might be off putting.
- Possible allergy to the material from which the diaphragm is made, or the spermicide.
- Increased risk of cystitis and urinary tract infections because secretions and bacteria are trapped in the vagina under the diaphragm for an increased length of time. Pressure on the bladder neck as a result of the diaphragm rim may also increase the risk of cystitis.

Contraindications

- Lack of tone of vaginal muscles.
- Genital tract bleeding.
- Congenital abnormalities of the vagina, e.g. septal wall defect.
- Previous toxic shock syndrome.
- Infection involving the vagina, cervix, or pelvic area.
- Reoccurring urinary tract infection.

Cap

The cap is made of rubber and is smaller than the diaphragm. It covers the cervix and is held in place by suction. Like the diaphragm, the failure rate is low if it is used correctly and with spermicide, i.e. between 92% and 96% effective (Belfield, 1999).

Three types of cervical cap are available:

- *Vault cap (Dumas cap)* – This cap is semi-circular, dome-shaped and shallow (Figure 8.5). Sizes range from 55–75 mm. This cap can be used by women

Figure 8.5 – Vault cap

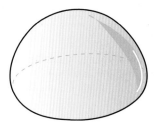

Figure 8.6 – Cervical cap

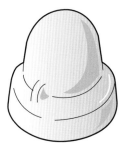

Figure 8.7 – Vimule cap

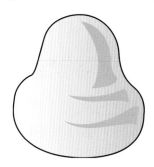

who have a shorter wider cervix and poor muscle tone. It is held in place by suction to the vaginal wall.

- *Cervical cap (Prentif cavity rim)* – This cap is shaped like a thimble and has a firm rim and adheres to the cervical wall by suction (Figure 8.6). It comes in four different sizes ranging from 22 to 31 mm. Women with a long, straight sided, symmetrical cervix will be able to use this cap.

- *Vimule cap* – The shape of this cap is a combination of the Vault and Cervical cap (Figure 8.7). It is dome shaped and wide at the sides. It is kept in position by suction to the vaginal wall. It can be used by women with an irregular shaped cervix. Sizes available are 42, 48, and 54 mm.

Figure 8.8 – IUD in position

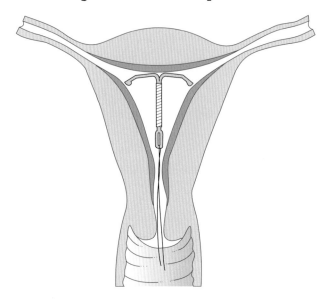

Contraindications, advantages, disadvantages, and instructions for use are the same as for the diaphragm. However, unlike the diaphragm, the cap can be used by women who have weak vaginal muscles. The cap may also be recommended to women who have suffered from cystitis when using a diaphragm as it does not cause an increase in urinary symptoms.

Intrauterine device

The intrauterine device (IUD), also known as the coil, is inserted through the cervix and positioned in the uterus (Figure 8.8).

Mode of action

- The IUD produces an inflammatory reaction, i.e. there is an increase in leucocytes in response to the IUD in the uterus. These leucocytes surround the IUD and destroy any sperm and possibly also the egg.

- The production of prostaglandins are stimulated in the uterus by the IUD. These stimulate the muscle of the womb to contract.

- The leucocytes also disrupt the endometrium and prevent implantation (Szarewski and Guillebaud, 2000).

IUDs used to be made of plastic but these devices are no longer available in the UK (although some women may still have them in situ). The more recent devices are made of copper and polyethylene and some contain silver. One of the newest IUDs (the Mirena) releases a low dose of the hormone – progestogen. Therefore, as well as having the same mode of action as outlined above, this device also has the same mechanism of action as the POP, i.e. it thickens cervical mucus, preventing the entry of sperm, thins the endometrium making implantation less likely, and can prevent ovulation.

The effectiveness of the IUD ranges from between 98% to almost 100% and the failure rate falls after the first year of use (Belfield, 1999). Advantages, disadvantages and contraindications of this method of contraception are described by Belfield (2000). These include the following:

Advantages

- It is a reliable, and convenient method of contraception.
- It is unobtrusive and is a long-term method of contraception.

Disadvantages

- Not a good choice for childless women under 25 years.
- The possibility of heavier, more painful periods and spotting between periods. The exception is the Mirena which makes periods lighter and less painful due to thinning of the endometrium.
- Expulsion of the IUD (this is most likely to occur during the first 3 months following insertion).
- The development of a pelvic infection. The risk of this is greatest during the first few weeks following insertion and is more likely in younger women who have not had children. Parity, age, sexual activity of the women and possibly corticosteroid therapy increase the risk of infection. However, infections tend to be prevented with the Mirena, as the cervical mucus is thickened, helping to prevent the entry of bacteria.
- There is a small risk of ectopic pregnancy.
- There is a small risk of perforation.
- If used within 5 days of unprotected sex, the IUD can be used as a method of postcoital contraception by preventing implantation.

Contraindications

The IUD is contraindicated in the following:

- women who experience heavy periods
- pelvic inflammatory disease (PID) or an untreated sexually transmitted disease (STD)
- known or suspected ectopic pregnancy
- uterine or cervical abnormalities
- bacterial endocarditis, severe infections or heart valve replacement

Spermicides

Spermicides should be used in conjunction with barrier methods, as their failure rate is high when used alone (Szarewski and Guillebaud, 2000). Spermicides are comprised of an active ingredient which destroys the sperm cell membrane and a carrier which enables the active ingredient to enter the vagina prior to intercourse. Spermicides also change the pH of the vagina making the environment hostile for sperm. Spermicides come in a variety of forms including creams, foams and pessaries and provide some protection against STDs including HIV (Belfield, 1999). Some individuals are allergic or sensitive to certain brands of spermicide. If this occurs, another brand should be used.

The Female Reproductive Cycle

The secretion of sex hormones by the reproductive system are controlled by the hypothalamus and pituitary gland. Puberty occurs due to a rise in sex hormone production. Hormones secreted by the hypothalamus stimulate the anterior pituitary gland to release Follicle Stimulating Hormone (FSH) and Luteinizing Hormone (LH). This results in ovulation, i.e. the release of a mature ovum, from the ovary, each month. At the same time, the uterus undergoes a number of changes in order to prepare for the implantation of a fertilised ovum and to be able to support a developing embryo. If fertilisation is to occur, both the ovarian and uterine cycles must be coordinated by the hormones of the reproductive tract. Conception will not result if ovulation fails to occur or, alternatively, the uterus does not prepare itself for implantation.

The menstrual cycle

The menstrual cycle can be divided into four stages (Rutishauser, 1994):

- *Menstruation* – Menstruation lasts for approximately between 4 and 6 days. During this period the lining of the endometrium is shed and about 40 ml of blood is lost. FSH and LH secretions from the anterior pituitary begin to increase during menstruation, causing the maturation of several ovarian follicles each containing an ovum.

- *Follicular phase* – At about day six of the menstrual cycle only one follicle continues to mature with the production of increasing quantities of oestrogen. The endometrium thickens and the cervical mucus, which extends through the cavity of the uterus and the uterine tubes, becomes thinner, stretchy, watery, and more alkaline. This aids the passage of sperm through the female reproductive tract.

- *Ovulatory phase* – The oestrogen, produced by the enlarging follicle, stimulates the growth of the follicle. During mid cycle, the oestrogen levels increase greatly, and this causes a surge in the secretion of LH from the anterior pituitary. The follicle bursts and ovulation occurs 34–38 h after this surge (Martini, 2000).

- *Luteal phase* – The cells of the ruptured follicle multiply and form a yellowish body called the corpus luteum. The corpus luteum produces progesterone and moderate amounts of oestrogen. High levels of progesterone are secreted for the next 7 days. This hormone prepares the body for pregnancy. The endometrium becomes increasingly vascularised, the endometrial glands enlarge and secrete a fluid containing sugars, amino acids and mucus, and the cervical mucus becomes thickened. If fertilisation does not occur, the corpus luteum degenerates approximately 1 week after ovulation. The production of oestrogen and progesterone is reduced over the 12 days following ovulation, by which time the corpus luteum is no longer functioning.

Figure 8.9 – Anterior pituitary hormone levels during the female reproductive cycle

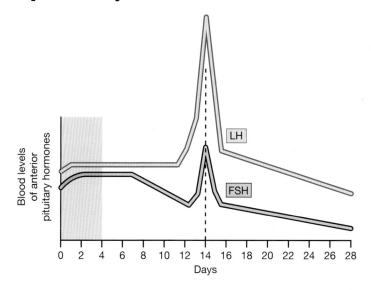

Figure 8.10 – Ovarian hormone levels during the female reproductive cycle

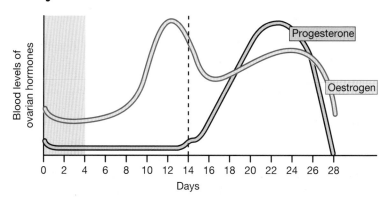

The endometrial lining becomes broken down and menstruation occurs. Oestrogen and progesterone concentrations fall further and FSH and LH, secreted from the anterior pituitary, begin a new cycle.

Oestrogen, progesterone, and progestogen

The functions of oestrogen, progesterone, and progestogen are described fully by Szarewski and Guillebaud (2000). The main functions identified include:

Oestrogen

The main activity of oestrogen is the development of the sex organs in the female, breast development, and fat and body hair distribution. The functions of oestrogen during the menstrual cycle include:

- Growth of the endometrium.
- The passage of the ovum into the uterine tube aided by the movement of the fimbrae towards the ovarian follicle.
- Contraction of the uterine tube transporting the ovum towards the uterus.
- Increase in sexual drive.
- Thinning of the cervical mucus facilitating the passageway of sperm.
- Increased suppleness of the vagina enabling it to expand during pregnancy and intercourse.
- Water retention.

Other important functions of oestrogen include the stimulation of bone and muscle growth and the production of hormones by the liver. These hormones include: sex hormone binding globulin, high-density lipoproteins, and blood clotting factors.

Sex hormone binding globulin

These hormones reduce the androgenic (male characteristics) effects of circulating testosterone and progestogens.

High-density lipoproteins

Complexes made of lipid (largely cholesterol) and protein. Their main function is to transport excess cholesterol from the peripheral tissues to the liver where they are stored or excreted in the bile.

Blood clotting factors

These are plasma proteins, which are necessary for normal coagulation.

Progesterone

Progesterone has an important role in the second half of the menstrual cycle. The functions of this hormone include:

- Continued preparation of the uterus for pregnancy.
- Stimulation of the breasts to produce milk (a combined role of prolactin and progesterone).
- Thickening of cervical mucus making it hard for sperm to penetrate.

Progesterone is destroyed in the stomach. Therefore, the contraceptive pill contains synthetic (artificial) progesterone called progestogen.

Progestogen

Progestogens are derived from the male sex hormone testosterone. Some of these preparations have a testosterone-like action and produce, for example acne and excess hair. Further adverse effects include:

- increased appetite and weight gain
- reduced sex drive
- increased risk of cardiovascular disease. This is caused by a reduction in high-density lipoproteins (which protect against atherosclerosis) and an

increase in low-density lipoproteins (which increase the risk of cardiovascular disease)

- a reduction in sex hormone binding globulin

Combined Oral Contraception (COC)

COC contains oestrogen and progestogen. Since its introduction 40 years ago, the oestrogen and progestogen levels have been greatly reduced to limit adverse effects. COCs in the UK contain either ethinyloestradiol or mestranol (synthetic oestrogens) and a progestogen. Progestogens available include desogestrel, gestodene, levonorgestrel, norethisterone acetate, ethynodiol diacetate, norgestrel, norethisterone, and norgestimate. Different types of COC are available. These include:

Monophasic pills

These identical tablets are taken for 21 consecutive days. Withdrawal bleeding then occurs during a 7 day break.

Phasic pills

The hormone content of each of these pills vary. Different strengths of pills are taken at varying points throughout the cycle. There is a 7 day break with these tablets.

Everyday pill

A pill is taken for each of the 28 days, i.e. there is no break. As 7 of the pills are inactive it is important to take them in the correct order. Phasic and monophasic varieties of these pills are available.

Whatever preparation is prescribed, the dose of oestrogen in the preparations available in the UK does not exceed 50 µg.

COC preparations:

Constituents	Trade Name
Combined standard strength	
7@ Norethisterone 500 µg & ethinyloestradiol 35 µg 14@ Norethisterone 1 mg & ethinyloestradiol 35 µg	BiNovum
Norethisterone 500 µg & ethinyloestradiol 35 µg	Brevinor
Norgestimate 250 µg & ethinyloestradiol 35 µg	Cilest
Levonorgestrel 250 µg & ethinyloestradiol 30 µg	Eugynon 30®
Gestodene 75 µg & ethinyloestradiol 30 µg	Femodene®
Gestodene 75 µg & ethinyloestradiol 30 µg plus 7 inactive	Femodene ED®
Combined low strength	
Gestodene 75 µg & ethinyloestradiol 20 µg	Femodette
Norethisterone acetate 1 mg & ethinyloestradiol 20 µg	Loestrin 20®

Combined standard strength

Norethisterone acetate 1.5 mg & ethinyloestradiol 30 μg	Loestrin 30®
6@ Levonorgestrel 50 μg & ethinyloestradiol 30 μg	Logynon®
5@ Levonorgestrel 75 μg & ethinyloestradiol 40 μg	
10@ Levonorgestrel 125 μg & ethinyloestradiol 30 μg	
6@ Levonorgestrel 50 μg & ethinyloestradiol 30 μg	Logynon ED®
5@ Levonorgestrel 75 μg & ethinyloestradiol 40 μg	
10@ Levonorgestrel 125 μg & ethinyloestradiol 30 μg	
plus 7 inactive	
Desogestrel 150 μg & ethinyloestradiol 30 μg	Marvelon®

Combined low strength

Desogestrel 150 μg & ethinyloestradiol 20 μg	Mercilon®

Combined standard strength

Levonorgestrel 150 μg & ethinyloestradiol 30 μg	Microgynon 30®
Levonorgestrel 150 μg & ethinyloestradiol 30 μg	Microgynon 30 ED®
plus 7 inactive	
Gestodene 75 μg & ethinyloestradiol 30 μg	Minulet®
Norethisterone 1 mg & ethinyloestradiol 35 μg	Norimin®

Combined high strength

Norethisterone 1 mg & mestranol 50 μg	Norinyl-1®
Levonorgestrel 250 μg & ethinyloestradiol 50 μg	Ovran®

Combined standard strength

Levonorgestrel 250 μg & ethinyloestradiol 30 μg	Ovran 30®
Levonorgestrel 150 μg & ethinyloestradiol 30 μg	Ovranette®
Norethisterone 500 μg & ethinyloestradiol 35 μg	Ovysmem®
7@ Norethisterone 500 μg & ethinyloestradiol 35 μg	Synphase®
9@ Norethisterone 1 mg & ethinyloestradiol 35 μg	
5@ Norethisterone 500 μg & ethinyloestradiol 35 μg	
6@ Gestodene 50 μg & ethinyloestradiol 30 μg	Triadene®
5@ Gestodene 70 μg & ethinyloestradiol 40 μg	
10@ Gestodene 100 μg & ethinyloestradiol 30 μg	
6@ Gestodene 50 μg & ethinyloestradiol 30 μg	Tri-Minulet®
5@ Gestodene 70 μg & ethinyloestradiol 40 μg	
10@ Gestodene 100 μg & ethinyloestradiol 30 μg	
6@ Levonorgestrel 50 μg & ethinyloestradiol 30 μg	Trinordiol®
5@ Levonorgestrel 75 μg & ethinyloestradiol 40 μg	
10@ Levonorgestrel 125 μg & ethinyloestradiol 30 μg	
7@ Norethisterone 500 μg & ethinyloestradiol 35 μg	TriNovum®
7@ Norethisterone 750 μg & ethinyloestradiol 35 μg	
7@ Norethisterone 1 mg & ethinyloestradiol 35 μg	

Mode of action

The combined pill has its effect by using several mechanisms. Mechanisms include:

- It causes inhibition of FSH. This suppresses follicular growth and the increased levels of oestrogen which stimulate the surge in LH.
- It changes the cervical mucus which impairs both the transport and penetration of sperm. Mucus becomes reduced, viscous and is no longer stretchy.
- It prevents implantation.
- It impairs sperm migration and transport of the ovum due to its effects on normal motility and secretions in the uterine tubes (Szarewski and Guillebaud, 2000).

The effectiveness of COCs ranges between 99.03% and 99.9% (Belfield, 1999).

The advantages, disadvantages, and contraindications for COC are outlined by Henry (2001). These include:

Advantages

- Extremely reliable
- Convenient to use
- Makes menstruation more regular and lessens blood loss
- Reduces pain during menstruation
- Reduces the risk of benign breast disease, endometriosis, ectopic pregnancy, and ovarian cysts
- Protects against PID, endometrial, and ovarian cancer

Disadvantages

- Requires compliance by the user
- Risk of
  - thromboembolism
  - heart disease
  - increased blood pressure
  - jaundice
  - gallstones
  - liver cancer
  - possible increase in the risk of breast and cervical cancer

Contraindications

- If pregnant or pregnancy is suspected.
- Uterine or vaginal bleeding of unknown origin.
- Those who have cardiovascular disease or, known risk factors, e.g. high blood lipid levels.

- A history of venous thrombosis.
- Blood disorders.
- High blood pressure.
- Migraine.
- Liver disease.
- Otosclerosis, i.e. hereditary ear disease leading to progressive deafness of the mechanical or conductive type.
- Over 35 years of age and a smoker.

Adverse effects

Women taking COC can suffer a number of minor adverse effects during the first few weeks that it is taken. The effects experienced are determined by the balance of oestrogen and progestogen in the preparation used. Bloating, nausea, breast tenderness, and weight gain are some of the adverse effects of oestrogen. Adverse effects of progestogen include acne, greasy hair, and depression.

Individuals who are at a greater risk of developing the serious adverse effects associated with COC include:

- Those with diabetes mellitus.
- Those with a close relative who has had a myocardial infarction or cerebrovascular accident.
- Those who are obese.
- Those who are older.
- Those who smoke.

The risks of cardiovascular disease and COC are discussed fully by Szarewski and Guillebaud (2000). Major issues include:

Venous disease and COC

As previously outlined, oestrogen causes an increase in blood clotting factors (although factors that cause clot breakdown are simultaneously produced) and therefore an increased tendency for the blood to clot, especially in the veins. There is a direct relationship between the dose of oestrogen in the pill and venous thrombosis. If the dose of oestrogen is reduced, the risk of thrombosis is decreased. The risk of venous thromboembolism (VTE) is also increased in the newer COC (containing desogestrel or gestodene, the newer third generation progestogens) compared to other COCs.

Arterial disease and COC

Oestrogen causes blood clotting factors to increase, as well as increasing the quantity of factors responsible for clot breakdown. Smoking prevents an increase in those factors which break down clots. Therefore, if a woman smokes and takes the pill, she is particularly at risk of developing a blood clot in an artery.

Fats are transported in the bloodstream in the form of lipoproteins (lipid-protein complexes). These complexes vary with regard to size, and their proportions of lipid and protein. High-density lipoproteins (HDLs) contain lipids, which are largely cholesterol. Their main function is to transport excess cholesterol from the peripheral tissues to the liver. From the liver, they are either stored or excreted in the bile. Low-density lipoproteins (LDLs), also contain cholesterol which is delivered to peripheral tissues. These lipoproteins from plaques in central vessels. Therefore, HDLs are occasionally referred to as good cholesterol as it is returning from the peripheral tissues and will not cause problems with the circulation. By contrast, LDLs are sometimes referred to as bad cholesterol (Martini, 2000).

Oestrogen and progestogen have an effect on lipoproteins. Oestrogen increases HDLs (lipoproteins which protect individuals against atherosclerosis) and decrease LDLs (lipoproteins which cause atherosclerosis). Oestrogen therefore protects against atherosclerosis. The older progestogen however, predisposes to atherosclerosis by increasing LDLs and decreasing HDLs. The negative effect of progestogen is compensated for by the positive effect of oestrogen in COC. Women taking the new progestogen pills have a lower risk of arterial disease.

Smoking has the same effect as progestogen, i.e. it raises LDLs and lowers HDLs. Therefore, women that smoke and take the COC are at an added risk of atherosclerosis. The compensatory effect of oestrogen over progestogen is lost. There is hardly any increase in the risk of arterial disease for young women (under 35) who do not smoke and use low dose pills. However, women who smoke must stop taking the pill at 35 years of age.

NB. There are a number of risk factors associated with arterial disease, e.g. family history, and abnormal blood lipid levels. It might be that the risk of atherosclerosis is increased if women who take the pill also have any of these risk factors.

Breast cancer
Findings from the Collaboration Group on Hormonal Factors in Breast Cancer (1996) identified that there is a slight risk of being diagnosed as having breast cancer whilst on the COC and for a period of 10 years following cessation. This risk is not associated with family history, dose, duration, or hormone type in the pill. Findings also identified that the breast cancers diagnosed in women taking the COC were clinically less advanced and less likely to have spread beyond the breast than in those not taking the COC.

Cervical cancer
A number of factors are thought to predispose to cervical cancer. The role of COC in increasing the risk of cervical cancer is not yet clear.

Medication and COC
Certain drugs can speed up the action of enzymes in the liver which destroy the hormones in the pill. This lessens the amount of hormone available for use by the body and therefore to prevent conception. Drugs that produce this effect include some of those used to treat epilepsy and tuberculosis. Rifampicin is a very strong enzyme inducer. In these circumstances the strength of the COC will be increased and additional contraceptive precautions required.

Broad-spectrum antibiotics, e.g. tetracyclines and penicillin, destroy bacteria living in the bowel. This affects COC as these bacteria normally convert the breakdown products of COC (i.e. the products which travel to the bowel following liver metabolism) into a useful form which are reabsorbed and used. Therefore, the oestrogen dose is lower than normal. This causes a risk of pregnancy. Additional contraceptive precautions should be taken during and following a course of antibiotics. However, if the pill is commenced during a long course of treatment with antibiotics, e.g. for acne, additional precautions are unnecessary as the bacteria will have become resistant (Belfield, 1999).

Progesterone-only-Pill

The POP contains the progestogens norethisterone, ethnodiol diacetate, or levonorgestrel. The dose of progestogen is lower than the dose used in the COC.

POP preparations:

Constituents	Trade Name
Etynodiol 500 µg	Femulen®
Norethisterone 350 µg	Micronor®
Levonorgestrel 30 µg	Microval®
Norgestrel 75 µg & levonorgestrel 37.5 µg	Neogest®
Levonorgestrel 30 µg	Norgeston®
Norethisterone 350 µg	Noriday®

Mode of action

The mechanism by which the POP works includes:

- The possible prevention of ovulation.
- The thickening of cervical mucus making sperm passage difficult.
- The thinning of the endometrial lining, preventing implantation.

The effectiveness of the POP ranges from 90% to 99% (Belfield, 1999). As a woman gets older and ovulation becomes less frequent, the effectiveness of the POP improves. The POP is a good choice for women over the age of 30 and the failure rate of the POP in women over 35 years is comparable to that of the COC. Therefore, it is recommended for women who smoke and need to stop taking the COC (Szarewski and Guillebaud, 2000).

The advantages, disadvantages, and contraindications of the POP are outlined by Everett (1997). These include:

Advantages

- The absence of oestrogen in this preparation, means it can be used in situations where the COC is not recommended.
- No increased risk of cardiovascular disease, venous thromboembolism, or hypertension.
- The POP can be continued before surgery.
- It is suitable for women who are breast feeding.

- It can be taken by patients with diabetes or by women who suffer from focal migraines.
- It may reduce dysmennorhoea and pre-menstrual symptoms.

Disadvantages

- The woman must remember to take the POP within 3 h of the time it was taken on the previous day. Failure to do this allows the cervical mucus to thin and allow the entry of sperm.
- It can cause menstrual irregularity.
- It can cause the development of functional ovarian cysts.
- There is a slight risk of ectopic pregnancy.
- Possible risk of breast cancer (as for COC).

Contraindications

- If an irregular menstrual cycle is unacceptable
- If the woman has been hospitalised for functional ovarian cysts
- Women who have had an ectopic pregnancy
- Undiagnosed uterine or vaginal bleeding
- Arterial disease
- Lipid abnormalities
- Recent trophoblastic disease
- If experienced serious adverse effects of COC not attributable to oestrogen
- Current liver disease, liver adenoma or cancer

Adverse effects

- Increase in weight
- Increase in blood pressure
- Tender breasts
- Nausea
- Acne
- Hirsutism (Galbraith et al., 1999)

Medication

The POP is effected by any medication that speeds up the action of liver enzymes and therefore breaks down progestogen (see COC).

Emergency Contraception

Emergency contraception or, postcoital contraception, is a safe and effective method of preventing pregnancy. There are three methods available, i.e. two hormonal preparations which are taken orally and a copper-containing IUD.

Emergency contraceptive preparations:

Constituents	Trade Name
Levonorgestrel 750 μg	Levonelle-2®
Norgestrel 500 μg (equivalent to levonorgestrel 250 μg) & ethinyloestradiol 50 μg	Schering PC4®

To be effective, hormonal preparations must be administered within 72 h of unprotected intercourse. The woman must initially take two high dose combined pills and then a further two pills 12 h later. This method works in the following ways:

- postpones ovulation
- acts on the endometrium and prevents implantation (Henry, 2001)

The effectiveness rate of this method of contraception ranges from 95% to 99% (Belfield, 1999). Principal indications for emergency contraception include:

- Unprotected sex
- Potential barrier method failures
- Potential pill failure when alternative methods have not been used or failed
- Potential IUD failure
- Risk of conception while advised to avoid pregnancy (Faculty of Family Planning and Reproductive Health Care, 2000)

Contraindications

Although the Summaries of Product Characteristics identify a number of conditions as precautions or contraindications for use, the World Health Organisation (WHO) (1998) considers established pregnancy as the only contraindication for the use of these preparations.

Adverse effects

- Nausea
- Vomiting (Faculty of Family Planning and Reproductive Health Care, 2000)

Medication

Enzyme inducing drugs such as Rifampicin reduce the efficacy of emergency contraception. In this situation women will be advised to increase the number of tablets taken.

Injectable progestogens

These products contain a higher dose of progestogen than the POP and provide a similar effect.

Injectable progestogen preparations:

Constituents	Trade Name
Medroxyprogesterone acetate 150 mg/ml	Depo-Provera®
Norethisterone enantate 200 mg/ml	Noristerat®

Mode of action

- Prevents ovulation
- Thickens cervical mucus
- Thins the endometrium preventing implantation

This method of contraception is nearly 100% effective.

Advantages, disadvantages, and contraindications of this method of contraception are described by Belfield (1999). These include the following:

Advantages

- There is an immediate effect following intramuscular injection within 5 days of menstruation.
- It is extremely effective and safe. A single injection lasts 8–12 weeks.
- It reduces pre-menstrual symptoms and painful periods.
- It is not linked to cardiovascular disease.
- It can be used whilst breast feeding.
- It has most of the non-contraceptive benefits of COC.

Disadvantages

- It can cause disturbances in menstruation.
- It can cause an increase in weight.
- It delays the return of fertility.
- Possible depression.
- It may be linked to osteoporosis.
- It is not possible to withdraw once administered.
- There is a risk of breast cancer similar to that of COC.

Contraindications

It should not be prescribed in women who

- might be pregnant
- may have breast or genital cancer
- suffer from vaginal or uterine bleeding of unknown cause
- have lipid abnormalities
- have had recent trophoblastic disease, active liver disease, liver adenoma or cancer

- have experienced serious adverse effects whilst taking COC which were not as a result of oestrogen
- experience progestogen sensitive migraine

Medication

It is affected by enzyme inducing drugs (*see* COC).

Preparations for Conditions of the Reproductive System

Bacterial vaginosis

The most common infectious cause of vaginitis is bacterial vaginosis. This condition is characterised by an alteration in the bacterial flora of the vagina. As opposed to a normal predominance of *Lactobacillus* species, there are high concentrations of anaerobic bacteria (Joesoef and Schmid, 2001). Only 50% of infected women are symptomatic.

A number of complications of pregnancy are associated with this condition (see Joesoef and Schmid, 2001 for a fuller discussion) and HIV acquisition and transmission is possibly enhanced by bacterial vaginosis (Schmid *et al.*, 2000).

Without treatment, symptoms might resolve or persist.

Preparations for the treatment of bacterial vaginosis:

- Clindamycin cream 2% (Dalacin® cream)
- Metronidazole vaginal gel 0.75% (Zidoval® vaginal gel)
- Metronidazole tablets

Contraindications, adverse effects, and nursing points for these preparations are discussed in Chapter 2.

Nursing Points

Although the cause of this condition is not fully understood, it has been identified that the likelihood of developing bacterial vaginosis is increased in women using an IUD and those taking oral contraceptives (Avonts *et al.*, 1990). New or multiple sexual partners (Barbone *et al.*, 1990; Avonts *et al.*, 1990; Hawes *et al.*, 1996), sexual debut at a young age (Hillier *et al.*, 1995), and douching (Hawes *et al.*, 1996) are other risk factors.

Antibiotic treatment is indicated in symptomatic women, women undergoing surgical procedures and some pregnant women (CEG, 1999). Oral metronidazole is the preferred choice (DTB, 1998; CEG, 1999). However, alternative treatments include intravaginal metronidazole gel or clindamycin cream. Following treatment, the condition will reoccur in about a third of women (Joesoef and Schmid, 2001).

Vulvovaginal candidiasis

Candida albicans is the yeast that is usually the infective micro-organism causing vulval candidiasis or thrush (*see* Chapter 4). Vulvovaginal candidiasis is often diagnosed on the basis of clinical symptoms alone. Symptoms include:

- vulval itching
- vulval soreness
- vaginal discharge
- pain during sexual intercourse (CEG, 1998)

A vaginal swab, taken for culture and sensitivity, will provide laboratory confirmation of the infection.

Preparations for the treatment of vulvovaginal candidiasis:

- Econazole nitrate pessary 150mg (Ecostatin 1®)
- Econazole nitrate pessaries 150 mg (Ecostatin® Pessaries)
- Econazole nitrate 150 mg pessaries with 1% cream (Ecostatin® Twinpack)
- Fenticonazole nitrate pessaries 200 mg (Lomexin®)
- Fluconazole 150 mg capsules (Diflucan®)
- Ovule (vaginal capsule) miconazole nitrate 1.2 g (Gyno-Daktarin 1®)
- Miconazole nitrate 100 mg pessaries with 2% cream (Gyno-Daktarin® combipack)
- Miconazole nitrate 2% intravaginal cream (Gyno-Daktarin® intravaginal cream)
- Miconazole nitrate 100 mg pessaries (Gyno-Daktarin®)
- Nystatin vaginal cream 100,000 units/4 g (Nystan®)
- Nystatin pessaries 100,000 units (Nystan®)

The preparations listed above are antifungal agents. Econazole, fenticonazole, fluconazole, and miconazole are all imidazoles. The actions, contraindications, adverse effects, and nursing points for these preparations and nystatin (also an antifungal agent) are described in Chapter 6. Further nursing points for the imidazoles, when used to treat vulvovaginal candidiasis are outlined below.

Nursing Points (Imidazoles)

Advice should include the avoidance of perfumed products which may cause local irritation. Loose fitting garments should also be worn. Imidazoles used for the treatment of vulvovaginal candidiasis are effective in short courses of 3–14 days depending upon the preparation used. It is important that the partners of sexually active individuals are also treated as the infection can be transmitted venerally (Galbraith *et al.*, 1999). Some of these preparations are supplemented with antifungal cream for vulvitis. If intravaginal agents are used, the absorption of these drugs are minimal and are associated with local reactions such as itching and burning. Systemic effects associated with these agents include headaches (Watson *et al.*, 2001). Systemic effects of oral preparations include gastro-intestinal effects and headaches (Watson *et al.*, 2001). Uncomplicated vulvovaginal candidiasis is treated equally as effectively with either oral or intravaginal agents (Watson *et al.*, 2001).

Dysmenorrhoea

Dysmenorrhoea is pain experienced in the lower abdomen or pelvic area during the onset of menstrual flow. It is commonly of 8–72 h duration. It is chronic and reoccurring, affecting most young women (Wilson and Farquhar, 2000). The aims of treatment are to relieve the pain with minimal adverse effects. It has been identified by Zhang and LiWan Po (1998) that non-steroidal anti-inflammatory drugs provide effective pain relief in the majority of women.

Preparations for the treatment of dysmenorrhoea:

- Ibuprofen granules 600 mg/sachet and syrup 100 mg/5 ml (Brufen®)
- Ibuprofen modified release tablets and capsules 800 mg (Brufen Retard®)
- Ibuprofen tablets 200 mg, 400 mg, 600 mg, 800 mg, and suspension 100 mg/1 ml (Brufen®)
- Oral contraceptives

The mode of action of these products, contraindications, adverse effects, and nursing points are addressed in this chapter and Chapter 3. Further nursing points are outlined below.

Nursing Points

The application of topical heat has been found to be effective in patients with dysmenorrhoea (Akin *et al.*, 2001).

The Penis

The penis is a tubular organ which allows the passage of urine to the exterior and the introduction of semen into the vagina during sexual intercourse. The penis is divided into three sections (Martini, 2000). These include:

- *The root* – this portion is fixed and attaches the penis to the body wall.
- *The body* – the tubular, movable portion that contains erectile tissue.
- *The glans* – the expanded distal end which encases the external urethral meatus.

The prepuce or foreskin is a fold of skin that surrounds the head (glans) of the penis. The body of the penis consists of three cylindrical columns of erectile tissue. The corpora cavernosa and the corpus spongiosum. This tissue includes blood vessels, elastic connective tissue, and smooth muscle. In the resting state, blood vessels are constricted and the smooth muscle is tense. This reduces blood flow into the erectile tissue. When the smooth muscle becomes relaxed, and the blood vessels become engorged, the penis becomes erect.

Balanitis

Tightening of the prepuce can prevent its retraction over the glans of the penis. This is called phimosis. Balanitis, i.e. inflammation of the glans, usually caused by a bacterial or fungal infection, is associated with phimosis. *Candida albicans* is the common causative organism. The glans becomes red and may itch, and a discharge may be present.

Preparations for the treatment of balanitis:

- Clotrimazole 1% and Betamethasone 0.05% (as dipropionate) cream (Lotriderm® cream)
- Clotrimazole 1% and Hydrocortisone 1% cream (Canesten HC® cream)
- Econazole 1% and Hydrocortisone 1% cream (Econacort® cream)
- Ketoconazole 2% cream (Nizoral® cream)
- Miconazole nitrate 2% and hydrocortisone 1% cream and ointment (Daktacort® cream and ointment)
- Nystatin 100,000 units/g, hydrocortisone 0.5% and chlorhexidine hydrochloride 1% cream, nystatin 100,000 units/g, hydrocortisone 0.5% and chlorhexidine acetate 1% ointment (Nystaform-HC®)
- Nystatin 100,000 units/g cream and ointment (Nystan®)
- Sulconazole nitrate 1% cream (Exelderm®)
- Nystatin 100,000 units/g, hydrocortisone 0.5%, benzalkonium chloride solution 0.2% and dimeticone '350' 10% (Timodine® cream)

The mode of action of these products, contraindications, adverse effects, and nursing points for these can be found in Chapter 6. Further discussion can also be found under vulvovaginal candidiasis.

Nursing Points

The foreskin should be retracted during the passing of urine. The glans should be regularly cleaned and kept dry (MCA, 2001). This may be all that is required and the condition often resolves itself. However, if treatment is required, a topical imidazole is the preparation of choice. Medical advice should be requested if this condition is severe or occurs frequently.

References

Akin MD, Weingand KW, Hengehold DA, *et al* (2001). Continuous topical heat was as effective as ibuprofen for dysmenorrhoea. *Evidenced Based Nursing* 4: October, 113.

Avonts D, Sercu M, Heyerick P, *et al* (1990). Incidence of uncomplicated genital infections in women using oral contraception or an intrauterine device: a prospective study. *Sex Transm Dis* 17: 23–29.

Barbone F, Austin H, Louv WC, Alexander WJ (1990). A follow-up study of methods of contraception, sexual activity, and rates of trichomoniasis, candidiasis, and bacterial vaginosis. *Am J Obstet Gynecol* 163: 510–514.

Belfield T (1999). FPA *Contraceptive Handbook* (3rd edn). London: Family Planning Association.

Bounds W (1994). Contraceptive efficiency of the diaphragm and cervical caps used in conjunction with a spermicide – a fresh look at the evidence. *The British Journal of Family Planning* 20: 84–87.

CEG (1998). National guidelines for the management of vulvovaginal candidiasis. *Clinical Effectiveness Group of the Association for Genitourinary Medicines and the Medical Society for the study of Venereal Diseases.* http://www.agum.org.uk/CEG/S19_thrush.html

CEG (1999). National guidelines on the management of bacterial vaginosis. *Clinical Effectiveness Group of the Association for Genitourinary Medicine and the Medical Society for the Study of Venereal Disease.* http://www.agum.org.uk/CEG/S16_bv.html

Collaboration Group on Hormonal factors in Breast cancer (1996). Breast cancer and hormonal contraceptives. *Contraception* 543 supplement.

DTB (1998). Managing urinary tract infection in women. *Drugs and Therapeutic Bulletin* 36: 30–32.

Everett S (1997). *Contraception and Family Planning*. London: Bailliere Tindall.

Faculty of Family Planning and Reproductive Health Care (2000). Emergency contraception: Recommendations for clinical practice. *Royal College of Obstetricians and Gynaecologists.* April 2000.

Galbraith A, Bullock S, Manias E, Hunt B, Richards A (1999). *Fundamentals of Pharmacology*. UK: Addison Wesley Longman Ltd.

Guillebaud J (1997) *Contraception Today* (3rd edn). London: Martin Dunitz Limited.

Hawes SE, Hillier SL, Benedetti J, *et al* (1996). Hydrogen peroxide-producing lactobacilli and acquisition of vaginal infections. *J Infect Dis* 174: 1058–1063.

Henry JA (2001). *The British Medical Association Concose Guide to Medicines and Drugs*. London: Dorling Kindersley.

Hillier SL, Nugent RP, Eschenback DA, *et al* (1995). Association between bacterial vaginosis and pre-term delivery of a low-birth-weight infant. *N Engl J Med* 333: 1737–1742.

Joesoef M, Schmid G (2001). Bacterial vaginosis. *Clinical Evidence* 5: 1075–1082.

Martini FH (2000). *Fundamentals of Anatomy and Physiology* (5th edn). New Jersey: Prentice Hall International.

MCA (2001). *Extended Prescribing of Prescription Only Medicines By Independent Nurse Prescribers*. London: MCA.

Rutishauser S (1994). *Physiology and Anatomy*. Edinburgh: Churchill Livingstone.

Schmid G, Markowitz L, Joesoef R, Koumans E (eds) (2000). Bacterial vaginosis and HIV infection. *Sex Trans Infect* 76: 3–4.

Szarewski A, Guillebaud J (2000). *Contraception: A User's Handbook* (2nd edn). Oxford: Oxford University Press.

Watson MC, Grimshaw JM, Bond CM, *et al* (2001). Review: Oral and intravaginal agents are equally effective for treatment of uncomplicated vulvovaginal candidiasis. *Evidenced Based Nursing*. Vol. 4. October, 112.

WHO (1998). *Emergency Contraception: A Guide to Service Delivery*. Geneva: WHO.

Wilson M, Farquhar C (2000). Dysmenorrhoea. *Clinical Evidence* March, 1255–1265.

Zhang WY, Li Wan Po A (1998). Efficacy of minor analgesics in primary dysmenorrhoea: a systematic review. *British Journal of Obstetrics and Gynaecology* 105: 780–789.

Chapter 9

Preparations for Problems and Minor Ailments of the Urinary System

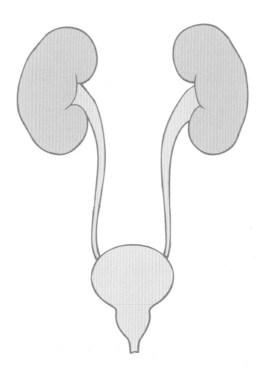

The Urinary System

The urinary system has two major functions. Firstly excretion, or the removal of waste products from body fluids, and secondly elimination, the removal of these wastes into the external environment. The urinary system includes the kidneys, the paired ureters, urinary bladder, and urethra (Figure 9.1). The kidneys are the site of urine production, whilst the ureters, bladder, and urethra form the conducting system for the transportation and storage of urine, prior to its elimination from the body. The term 'lower urinary tract' refers to the urethra and bladder, whilst the term 'upper urinary tract' refers to the ureters and renal pelves of the kidney. Although the kidneys perform all the vital functions of the urinary system, problems with the conducting system can have direct and immediate effects on renal function (Martini and Welch, 2001).

Figure 9.1 – Urinary system

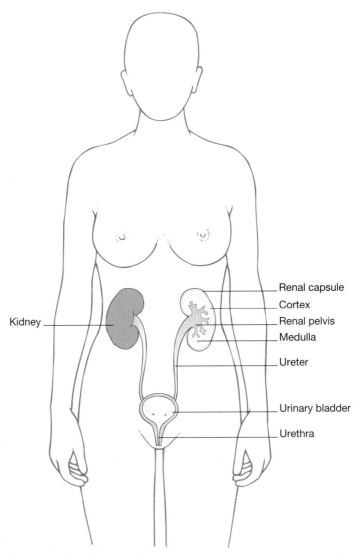

Kidney

Renal capsule
Cortex
Renal pelvis
Medulla
Ureter
Urinary bladder
Urethra

Uncomplicated, lower urinary tract infection

The nurse prescriber is able to prescribe medication for uncomplicated, lower urinary tract infection in women. An uncomplicated urinary tract infection is one where the individual has an anatomically and physiologically normal urinary tract, normal renal function, and there is no associated disorder which impairs defence mechanisms (Davison *et al.*, 1999). In women, the urethra is short and in close proximity to the vagina and rectum. This offers little protection against the entry of micro-organisms into the bladder from these areas. The main risk factors for uncomplicated urinary tract infections are sexual intercourse, personal or family history of urinary tract infection, and use of the contraceptive diaphragm plus spermicide (DTB, 1998). Urinary tract infections are also more common during pregnancy. Normal changes in the functioning of the urinary tract that occur during pregnancy, predispose to these infections (Porth, 1994). In 70% of cases, *Escherichia coli* is the causative organism (Gruneberg, 1994) with the remaining 30% being caused by *Proteus mirabilis*, *Klebsiella pneumoniae*, and *Staphylococcus saprophyticus*.

Symptoms of lower urinary tract infection, which is commonly cystitis, include lower abdominal discomfort, dysuria, and frequency and urgency of micturition. Cloudy or foul-smelling urine, haematuria and confusion (especially in the elderly) may also occur.

Diagnosis can be made based on the patient's history and clinical signs and without the need for urine culture. Dipstick urine tests however, are available in general practice, and these are good indicators of the presence of urinary tract infection (Ditchburn and Ditchburn, 1990). The leucocyte esterase test detects pus cells in urine, while bacteria in the urine that reduce nitrate to nitrite can be detected by the nitrate reductase test (Dawson and Whitfield, 1997).

Children and men with suspected or confirmed urinary tract infection and people with suspected upper urinary tract infection (pyelonephritis), require medical assessment by a physician. The DoH (2000) also indicates medical assessment for those patients with frank haematuria, or those patients over 50 years of age with microscopic haematuria.

Management

Patients should be encouraged to drink 3 l of fluid a day in order to keep the urine dilute. Making the urine alkaline by giving sodium bicarbonate or potassium citrate may make urination less painful (Blandy, 1998). Cranberry juice and other cranberry products have also been suggested to inhibit the adherence of bacteria to mucosal cells (Beachy, 1981), and have been recommended to patients with urinary tract infection. Busuttil-Leaver (1996) identifies some of the potential effects of cranberry juice but more research appears to be required regarding its effectiveness and role in prevention of urinary tract infection (Cooper and Jepson, 2001). Oral antibiotics may also be prescribed.

Preparations for the treatment of urinary tract infection:

- Amoxicillin
- Nitrofurantoin
- Trimethoprim

The mode of action, contraindications, and adverse effects for each of these drugs is described in Chapter 2.

The first line antibiotics for treatment of cystitis are trimethoprim or nitrofurantoin. Winstanley *et al.* (1997) indicate that trimethoprim is effective against 70% of urinary pathogens.

A 3-day course of an oral antibiotic is usually used to treat uncomplicated cystitis (Norrby, 1990). If symptoms do not respond to empirical antibiotics within 2–3 days, a urine sample should be obtained for culture and sensitivity testing (DTB, 1998).

In pregnancy, all urinary tract infections should be treated, and eradication of the infection should be confirmed by a urine culture test. Nitrofurantoin or a cephalosporin are recommended for blind treatment whilst waiting for the results of a urine culture and sensitivity test. Urine culture is essential in pregnant women with urinary tract infection. Co-amoxiclav, trimethoprim, tetracyclines, and quinolones are not recommended for use in pregnancy.

Nursing Points

In addition to the information already given regarding increasing fluid intake and the use of alkalising agents, mild analgesia (aspirin, paracetamol) may be required and local pain relief using a heat pad may be beneficial (Fillingham and Douglas, 1997).

Advice about preventing future infection includes maintaining an adequate fluid intake, not allowing the bladder to get overfull, ensuring that the bladder is completely emptied when voiding, and emptying the bladder after sexual intercourse.

There is no evidence to suggest that changing some behaviours, such as wearing synthetic underwear or tight underclothes, or using bath additives has any effect on the recurrence of urinary tract infections (Leiner, 1995).

Catheter patency problems

Many nurse prescribers will be involved in the care of patients with long term, indwelling, urinary catheters. Several complications are associated with the use of catheters, including catheter blockage, catheter encrustation, inflammatory reactions, trauma, urine infection, pain, and discomfort (Winn, 1998). Kunin *et al.* (1987) report that approximately 50% of all patients with an indwelling catheter are prone to catheter blockage which occurs secondary to encrustation. In addition, blocked catheters may cause bypassing of urine or retention of urine.

Encrustation

In alkaline conditions, ammonium phosphate, calcium phosphate or magnesium phosphate may precipitate from the urine and collect on the tip or around the eyes or the balloon of the catheter. In addition, infected urine is also more likely to lead to encrustation. The presence of bacteria such as *Proteus*, *Klebsiella*, and *Pseudomonas* specifically encourage the process of encrustation (Getliffe, 1997). It is the release of urease enzyme from these micro-organisms which breaks down urea to release ammonia and hydrogen ions, hence causing an increase in urine alkalinity.

The presence of a biofilm on the surface of the catheter also increases the risk of infection, encrustation, and associated problems (Ramsey, 1989). A biofilm is a collection of micro-organisms and their products on a solid surface (Wilson, 1998).

Bacteria within the biofilm produce a glycocalyx or thick coat of polysaccharides. This coat protects the micro-organisms from the body's natural defence mechanisms and antimicrobial drugs.

Catheter material

The type of catheter material may have some effect on the development of encrustation and development of a biofilm. Winn (1998) reports the results of several studies that indicate that all-silicone catheters are less likely to become encrusted than silicone-coated, Teflon-coated and latex catheters over 14 days. Hydrogel-coated catheters appear to be as resistant to encrustation as all-silicone catheters over a period up to 18 weeks. In addition, hydrogel-coated catheters are less prone to bacterial adherence than silicone catheters. However, the ideal catheter, resisting encrustation and biofilm development, is not yet available, and nurses need to be aware of the specific characteristics of products in order to make an informed choice about which appliance to choose for their patient.

Catheter life

Getliffe (1996) suggests that by observing and recording the length of time that a patient's catheter continues to function before becoming blocked, will reveal a pattern of 'catheter life'. It should then be possible to plan future recatheterisations before blockage has a chance to occur.

In addition, the reduction of urine alkalinity by consumption of cranberry juice may assist in prolonging catheter life. The resulting acidification of urine may prevent infection and encrustation. The need for further research into the effectiveness of cranberry juice and cranberry products was mentioned earlier in this chapter. If a patient experiences no problem with blockage, the catheter needs to be changed approximately once in 3 months, if all-silicone, silicone-coated or hydrogel-coated. Latex catheters require changing every 6 weeks in most instances. However, frequent blocking requires either recatheterisation, which can be painful if it is being done often, or the use of an appropriate bladder washout solution to attempt to relieve the obstruction.

Preparations for catheter maintenance:

- Chlorhexidene 0.02% (Uro-Tainer Chlorhexidene®, Uriflex C®)
- Mandelic Acid (Uro-Tainer Mandelic Acid®)
- Sodium Chloride 0.9% (Uro-Tainer Sodium Chloride®, Uriflex S®)
- 'Solution G' (Uro-Tainer Suby G®, Uriflex G®)
- 'Solution R' (Uro-Tainer Solution R®, Uriflex R®)

Chlorhexidene 0.02% solution is available for mechanical cleansing and prevention of contamination by bacteria, specifically *E. coli* and *Klebsiella*. It is usually ineffective against most species of *Pseudomonas*. Mandelic acid 1% aids acidification in order to prevent growth of urease-producing bacteria, as well as mechanically cleansing the catheter and bladder. Sodium chloride 0.9% will aid small blood clot removal and tissue debris that may be present. 'Solution G' specifically prevents encrustation and crystallisation. 'Solution R' is recommended for prevention of encrustation and crystallisation when 'Solution G' has been unsuccessful.

Contraindications

None identified.

Adverse effects

Chlorhexidene 0.02% may irritate the bladder causing burning and haematuria. It should be discontinued in these circumstances.

Nursing Points

The use of a catheter maintenance solution requires the breaking of a closed drainage system. Aseptic technique must, therefore, be performed when administering a solution. A new drainage bag should be connected following the procedure. Hands should be washed thoroughly before and after the procedure. The solution should be warmed to body temperature before instillation. Gravity is used to instil the solution and not active flushing. Ideally, bladder washouts should only be used when absolutely necessary. However prophylactic washouts in patients with frequently blocked catheters, may extend the catheter life.

Patients and/or their carers can be taught to administer a catheter patency solution. Patient or carer assessment is essential in order to establish that they have the manual dexterity and ability to undertake their own catheter management. A planned teaching programme will be necessary to help them develop confidence and competence in catheter care (Getliffe, 1996). Patients should be encouraged to maintain an adequate fluid intake to reduce the irritant effects of concentrated urine and maintain urine flow. An intake of 1.5–2.0 l per day is recommended. However, a high fluid intake cannot prevent or reduce infection, but diuresis may assist in voiding micro-organisms from the bladder. If patients wish to consume cranberry juice, then the nurse should attempt to monitor its effects on the patient. No more than 1 l per day should be consumed, as an excessive intake may lead to uric acid stone formation. Patients with irritable bowel syndrome may develop diarrhoea. In addition, cranberry juice is rather expensive and some individuals will dislike its taste.

References

Beachy EH (1981). Bacterial adherence; adhesion receptor interactions mediating the attachment of bacteria to mucosal surfaces. *Journal of Infectious Diseases* 143: 325–345.

Blandy J (1998). *Lecture Notes on Urology* (5th edn). Oxford: Blackwell Science.

Busuttil-Leaver R (1996). Cranberry juice. *Professional Nurse* May, 11(8): 525–526.

Cooper B, Jepson R (2001). Recurrent cystitis in non-pregnant women. *Clinical Evidence* 5: 1338–1345.

Davison AM, Cumming AD, Swainson CP, Turner N (1999). Infections of the kidney and urinary tract. In: Haslett C, Chilvers ER, Hunter JAA, Boon NA (eds). *Davidson's Principles and Practice of Medicine* (18th edn). Edinburgh: Churchill Livingstone.

Dawson C, Whitfield H (1997). *ABC of Urology*. London: BMJ.

DoH (2000). *Referral Guidelines for Suspected Cancer*. DoH.

Ditchburn RK, Ditchburn RS (1990). A study of microscopical and chemical tests for the rapid diagnosis of urinary tract infections in general practice. *British Journal of General Practice* 40: 406–408.

DTB (1998). Managing urinary tract infection in women. *Drug and Therapeutics Bulletin* 36(4): 30–32.

Fillingham S, Douglas J (1997). *Urological Nursing*. (2nd edn). London: Balliere Tindall.

Getliffe K (1996). Care of urinary catheters. *Nursing Standard* 11(11): 47–50.

Getliffe K (1997). Catheters and catheterisation. In: Getliffe K, Dolman M (eds). *Promoting Continence: A Clinical and Research Resource*. London: Balliere Tindall.

Gruneberg RN (1994). Changes in urinary pathogens and their antibiotic sensitivities, 1971–1992. *J Antimicrobial Chemotherapy* 33(Suppl. 8): 1–8.

Kunin CM, Chin QF, Chambers S (1987). Formation of encrustations on indwelling urinary catheters in the elderly: a comparison of different types of catheter materials in 'blockers' and 'non-blockers'. *Journal of Urology* 138(4): 899–902.

Leiner S (1995). Recurrent urinary tract infections in otherwise healthy adult women. *Nurse Practitioner* 20(2): 448–456.

Martini FH, Welch K (2001). *Applications Manual for Fundamentals of Anatomy and Physiology* (5th edn). Upper Saddle River: Prentice-Hall.

Norrby, SR (1990). Short-term treatment of uncomplicated lower urinary tract infections in women. *Rev Infect Dis* 12: 458–467.

Porth CM (1994). *Pathophysiology: Concepts of Altered Health States* (4th edn). Philadelphia: JB Lippincott.

Ramsey J (1989). Biofilms, bacteria and bladder catheters – A clinical study. *British Journal of Urology* 64: 395–398.

Wilson M (1998). Infection control. *Professional Nurse Study Supplement* February, 13(5): S10–S13.

Winn C (1998). Complications with urinary catheters. *Professional Nurse Study Supplement* February, 13(5): S7–S10.

Winstanley TG, Limb DI, Eggington R, Hancock F (1997). A 10 year survey of the microbial susceptibility of urinary tract isolates in the UK: the Microbe base project. *J Antimicrob Chemother* 40: 591–594.

Chapter 10

Preparations for Problems and Minor Ailments of the Sense Organs

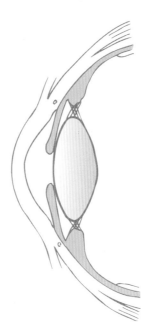

The Eye

In order to manage and prescribe for problems affecting the eye, the nurse prescriber must be familiar with the accessory and protective structures of the eye.

The eyelids or palpebrae, are a continuation of the skin, which through their continual blinking movements keep the surface of the eye lubricated and free from dust and debris. The two eyelids are connected at the medial canthus and lateral canthus, and are separated by a gap called the palpebral fissure (Figure 10.1). The eyelashes are robust hairs along the margins of the eyelids which prevent foreign particles from reaching the surface of the eye. Along the inner margin of the eyelid are modified sebaceous glands called tarsal glands (Meibomian glands), which secrete a lipid-rich product that prevents the eyelids sticking together. The lacrimal caruncle found at the medial canthus, also produces thick secretions.

The epithelium covering the inner surfaces of the eyelids and the outer surface of the eye is the conjunctiva (Figure 10.2). The palpebral conjunctiva covers the inner

Figure 10.1 – External features of the eye

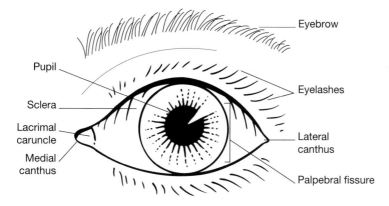

Figure 10.2 – Anatomy of the eye

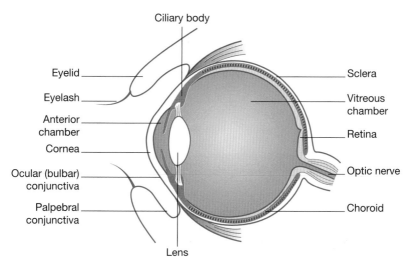

surface of the eyelids and the ocular conjunctiva (bulbar conjunctiva) covers the anterior surface of the eye, extending to the cornea. A constant supply of fluid washes over the surface of the eyeball, keeping the ocular conjunctiva and cornea clean and moist. Goblet cells assist the accessory glands in providing a lubricant that prevents friction and drying of the opposing conjunctival surfaces (Martini, 2001).

Blepharitis

Blepharitis is inflammation of the margin of the eyelid. There are two main types: staphylococcal and seborrhoeic. Staphylococcal blepharitis is due to infection by *Staphylococcus aureus*, or *Staphylococcus epidermidis*, or coagulase-negative staphylococci. Seborrhoeic blepharitis is usually associated with the presence of *Pityrosporium ovale*. Often both types are present causing mixed infection (Sullivan *et al.*, 1999). Seborrhoea of the ears, brows and scalp (*see* Chapter 6) is frequently associated with seborrhoeic blepharitis.

Symptoms may be intermittent and include sore eyelids, irritation, itching of the lid margins and a gritty sensation. The patient may also present with a chalazion (stye), which is common in this condition. Scales are seen clinging to the lashes of the upper and lower lids, the lid margins appear inflamed and the tarsal gland orifices may be blocked. Inflammation of the conjunctiva may be present.

Management
Khaw and Elkington (1999) identify four main aspects of treatment:

1. The lids should be kept clean by using cotton buds dipped in warm water. The addition of baby shampoo may assist in removing crusty and coagulated lipid.

2. Infection should be treated using an antibiotic ointment that is smeared onto the eyelid margin.

3. Tears may need to be replaced using artificial tears.

4. Severe cases and those with sebaceous gland dysfunction may require oral tetracycline. This, however, is not within the remit of the nurse prescriber. Patients should be referred to a physician.

Treatment may be required for up to 1 month after inflammation has settled. Patients not responding to treatment must be referred to a physician for medical assessment and exclusion of other pathology.

Preparations for the treatment of blepharitis:

- Chloramphenicol eye ointment (Chloromycetin®)

The reader should consult Chapter 2 for the mode of action, contraindications, adverse effects, and nursing points related to this antibiotic.

Nursing Points

The patient or carer may need instruction on how to clean the eye and the application of the eye ointment.

Blurring of vision may follow application of the eye ointment, together with a possible burning or stinging sensation.

Eye ointment is usually applied 3–4 times daily.

Conjunctivitis

Conjunctivitis is inflammation of the conjunctiva. It is the most common eye disease worldwide, and is one of the most common causes of 'red eye' presenting to the general practitioner. There are many causes of conjunctivitis, and the nurse prescriber is able to treat both allergic conjunctivitis and infective conjunctivitis. These will be discussed separately.

Allergic conjunctivitis

Allergic conjunctivitis is commonly associated with allergic reactions such as hayfever (allergic rhinitis) or asthma, or there may have been recent contact with chemicals such as eye make-up, or the use of eye drops. Some contact lens wearers develop conjunctivitis. This may be improved by a change in contact lens solution.

The patient may complain of severe itching, moderate tearing, and redness of the eyes. On examination the conjunctiva is likely to be oedematous (chemosis) with a clear discharge. A 'cobblestone'-like appearance under the upper lid may be present. These round swellings or papillae are due to oedema. A minority of patients will be severely affected by allergic conjunctivitis. These are mainly highly atopic children and young adults suffering from eczema and/or asthma, and they will require careful supervision under the care of a physician (Tullo and Donnelly, 1995).

Management

Topical treatments include antihistamines and mast cell stabilisers. Oral antihistamines may also be necessary (*see* Chapter 5 for further details). Topical corticosteroids should only be used with regular opthalmological supervision, due to the risk of steroid-induced cataracts and glaucoma (Khaw and Elkington, 1999).

Preparations for the treatment of allergic conjunctivitis:

- Azelastine eye drops (Optilast®)
- Levocabastine eye drops (Livostin®)
- Lodoxamide eye drops (Alomide®)
- Nedocromil sodium eye drops (Rapitil®)
- Sodium cromoglicate eye drops

Azelastine and Levocabastine are topical antihistamines. The reader should consult Chapter 5 for the mode of action, contraindications, adverse effects, and nursing points related to antihistamines.

Nedocromil and sodium cromoglycate are both described as 'mast cell stabilisers'. Mast cells are connective tissue cells, which when stimulated or activated, release chemicals such as histamine and prostaglandins, responsible for initiating the inflammatory response. Activation and the subsequent rupture or degranulation of mast cells present in the eye, results in the release of inflammatory mediators responsible for the symptoms of allergic conjunctivitis. These drugs prevent degranulation and therefore, the inflammatory response. However, their mode of action is not fully understood.

Contraindications

None listed for topical application of either drug.

Adverse effects

Both drugs may cause transient burning or stinging on application.

Nursing Points

The patient or carer may need instruction on instillation of the eye drops.

Blurring of vision may follow application of the eye drops/ointment, together with possible burning or stinging sensation.

Soft contact lenses should not be worn during treatment with eyedrops due to possible absorption of the medication or preservatives.

If the causative allergen is not known, discussion with the patient may assist in establishing the cause.

Infective conjunctivitis

Infective conjunctivitis may be due to bacterial or viral infection. In both cases, the eye appears red with engorged conjunctival vessels.

Bacterial infection is most commonly due to infection by Staphylococcus species, followed by infection from *Streptococcus pneumoniae* and *Haemophilus influenzae*. The patient usually has a purulent exudate in one eye and sticky lids on waking. The infection usually starts in one eye and is spread to the other eye via the hand. It may be spread from person to person by fomites.

Viral conjunctivitis is more common than bacterial conjunctivitis, and usually due to highly infectious adenoviruses. This type of conjunctivitis usually occurs in epidemics. The patient will complain of gritty eyes with a watery discharge. They may also have a sore throat and fever, associated with an upper respiratory tract infection. The infection may persist for weeks, much longer than in bacterial conjunctivitis. A number of viral serotypes may cause a severe keratoconjunctivitis and on occasion, lasting visual disturbance due to characteristic round corneal lesions (Tullo and Donnelly, 1995). Photophobia and discomfort may be problematic if this arises.

Management

This involves preventing spread of infection to the other eye and to other individuals. In addition, topical antibiotics are usually prescribed empirically. They will hasten clinical improvement in bacterial conjunctivitis (Chung and Cohen, 2000) and provide symptomatic relief and prevent secondary bacterial infection for those with viral conjunctivitis (Khaw and Elkington, 1999). Topical chloramphenicol has a broad spectrum of activity and is the drug of choice for superficial infections. It is the only topical antibiotic possibly associated with serious systemic adverse effects (aplastic anaemia). However, Chung and

Cohen (2000) report no good evidence about the magnitude of this risk for chloramphenicol versus other topical antibiotics.

Preparations for the treatment of infective conjunctivitis:

- Chloramphenicol eye drops and eye ointment (Chloromycetin®, Sno Phenicol®, Minims® Chloramphenicol)
- Fusidic acid eye drops (Fucithalmic®)

The reader should consult Chapter 2 for the mode of action, contraindications, adverse effects, and nursing points related to these antibiotics.

Nursing Points

Strict hygiene measures are of utmost importance in preventing spread of infection. Patients should be advised to use their own flannel, towel, and pillow case. Where possible, they should administer their own treatment, washing their hands before and after touching the eye.

The patient or carer may need instruction on how to clean the eye and the instillation of the eye drops/ointment.

Blurring of vision may follow application of the eye drops/ointment, together with a possible burning or stinging sensation.

Eye drops are usually applied as one drop every 2 h, then reducing the frequency as infection is controlled. They should be continued for 48 h after healing. Eye ointment is usually applied at night if eye drops are being used during the day, or 3–4 times daily if used alone.

Contact lens should not be worn whilst treatment is undertaken and eye make-up should be avoided.

Lack of response to treatment requires medical assessment.

The Ear

The ear is divided into three main parts: the external ear, middle ear, and inner ear (Figure 10.3). The external ear consists of the pinna, external auditory meatus (ear canal) and tympanic membrane (eardrum).

The pinna is the large, skin-covered flap of cartilage which collects sound waves and channels them into and down the external auditory meatus. It also protects the opening of the external auditory meatus. In the adult, the external auditory meatus is approximately 2.5 cm long and its entrance is guarded by fine hairs.

The skin lining this canal contains wax-secreting ceruminous glands, which are modified sebaceous glands. The earwax or cerumen, consists of the secretion of the ceruminous glands, together with desquamated epithelial cells shed from the skin lining the canal, and variable amounts of hair. It functions to trap foreign objects and insects, and to slow the growth of micro-organisms in the ear canal. The presence of immunoglobulins and lysozymes, together with the skin of the ear being approximately pH 6.0, is thought to assist in defence against invading

Figure 10.3 – Anatomy of the ear

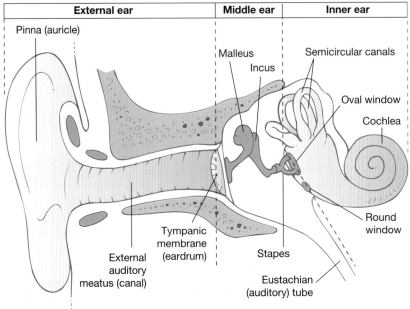

micro-organisms (Li Wan Po, 1990). Cerumen also prevents the skin of the external ear from drying out. Both the hairs and earwax will reduce the chance of airborne particles from reaching the inner part of the ear canal where they may accumulate and interfere with hearing.

The ear canal ends at the tympanic membrane which stretches across the entrance to the middle ear.

The tympanic membrane, a thin, semi-transparent membrane, vibrates when struck by sound waves that have been directed along the ear canal. The air-filled middle ear then transfers the vibratory movements of the tympanic membrane to the fluid of the inner ear. Three small bones (the *malleus*, *incus*, and *stapes*), also called the auditory ossicles, facilitate the transfer of vibrations through the middle ear. The stapes is attached to the oval window which bows in and out as the stapes moves back and forth. Movement of the oval window causes waves to occur in the fluid of the cochlea. A further series of events in the inner ear ultimately leads to the interpretation of sound by the central nervous system. For a fuller discussion of this process the reader should refer to Martini (2001).

Conductive Hearing Loss

There are several reasons why sound waves may not be transmitted to the inner ear. These include blockage of the external auditory meatus, infection of the middle ear, perforation of the tympanic membrane and immobilisation of one or more of the auditory ossicles. These conditions in the external and middle ear prevent the normal transfer of vibrations from the tympanic membrane to the oval window. This results in difficulties with hearing, referred to as conductive hearing loss (conductive deafness).

Earwax

The most common cause of partial, conductive hearing loss is the accumulation of earwax in the external auditory meatus. Normally, wax migrates naturally to the outside of the external meatus but this process may be hindered. If ear hairs are tough (as in elderly males), or if the patient attempts to clean the ears by poking a cotton wool bud down the canal, the wax may simply be pushed in the wrong direction. Not infrequently, the wax may become impacted in the canal, where, over time, it becomes hard (Serra *et al.*, 1986). As earwax is a normal body secretion with protective functions, it should only be removed if it is causing hearing problems or interfering with a view of the eardrum on examination. Excessive wax or blockage by wax may be treated by instilling ear drops to soften the wax, or by ear syringing with warm water. Burton and Mogg (2001) report that wax softeners are better than no treatment at completely removing ear wax without syringing. In addition, they report that there is no consistent evidence that any one type of wax softener is superior to the others.

Preparations for the treatment of excessive earwax:

- Almond oil ear drops
- Olive oil ear drops

These preparations may be referred to as ceruminolytics as they soften and loosen excessive or impacted wax (cerumen).

Contraindications

The nurse prescriber should avoid prescribing ear drops to: patients with a history of ear disease, to all cases of earache, and patients complaining of dizziness or an ear discharge. It is advisable to refer the patient to their physician for further assessment.

Adverse effects

These are not common. Minor skin irritation may occur.

Nursing Points

Ear drops should be warmed prior to instillation. This is best achieved by holding the bottle of oil in the hand for 5–10 min, allowing the temperature of the preparation to rise to body temperature. The patient should lie with the affected ear uppermost. A reasonable amount of oil is introduced into the ear and the patient should remain in the same position for 5–10 min to enable softening of the wax. The patient or carer will need to be instructed about administration of the ear drops. If ear syringing is required, following wax softening using ear drops, it should only be undertaken by a proficient practitioner trained in the procedure.

Mechanical probing of the ears with implements such as cotton buds, hair pins, and matchsticks should be discouraged. This only serves to enhance blockage by wax and could possibly perforate the eardrum. Baxter (1983) recommends that ceruminolytics are safer than cotton buds.

Otitis externa

Otitis externa is inflammation of the external ear, affecting the pinna and/or external auditory meatus. It may vary in severity from a mild eczemoid dermatitis to severe cellulitis. It may be caused by infectious agents or materials contained in earphones or earrings (contact dermatitis). Most external ear infections tend to be bacterial, with occasional secondary fungal infection. Predisposing factors can include moisture in the ear canal after swimming or bathing, trauma resulting from scratching or attempts to clean the ear, and allergic dermatitis (Porth, 1994). Manifestations include redness, scaliness, narrowing of the ear canal because of swelling, itching, pain, discharge, and hearing loss.

Management

The external auditory meatus should be cleaned, and discharge and debris be removed. Many cases recover after thorough cleansing by dry mopping, gentle syringing or suction. If infection is present, a topical antibacterial may be prescribed. This should only be used for a week, as excessive use may result in fungal infection. Sensitivity to the drug or solvent may occur and resistance to antibiotics may occur with prolonged use.

Solutions containing an antibiotic and corticosteroid are used when there is infection, inflammation, itching, and eczema.

The Committee on Safety of Medicines (CSM) has issued a reminder that treatment with a topical aminoglycoside antibiotic (neomycin, framycetin, gentamycin) is contraindicated in patients with tympanic perforation due to risk of ototoxicity.

Oral antibiotics may not be prescribed by the nurse prescriber and, patients who are systemically unwell and where there is evidence of spread of infection, should be referred to a physician.

Pain relief should be provided with appropriate analgesia (*see* Chapter 3).

Preparations for the treatment of otitis externa:

- Betamethasone and Neomycin drops (Betnesol-N®, Vista-Methasone N®)
- Betamethasone Sodium Phosphate drops (Betnesol®, Vista-Methasone®)
- Flumetasone Pivalate Ear Drops (Locorten-Vioform®)
- Gentamicin drops (Garamycin®, Genticin®)

- Hydrocortisone and Gentamicin drops (Gentisone HC®)
- Hydrocortisone and Neomycin drops and ointment (Neo-Cortef®)
- Prednisolone and Neomycin drops (Predsol-N®)
- Prednisolone Sodium Phosphate drops (Predsol®)
- Triamcinolone and Neomycin ear drops (Audicort®)

The reader should consult Chapter 2 for the mode of action, contraindications, adverse effects, and nursing points related to antibiotics. They should consult Chapter 6 for the mode of action, contraindications, adverse effects and nursing points related to topical corticosteroids.

References

Baxter P (1983). Association between the use of cotton tipped swabs and cerumen plugs. *British Medical Journal*, 287: 1260.

Burton M, Mogg E (2001). Wax in ear. *Clinical Evidence* 5: 370–375.

Chung C, Cohen E (2000). Bacterial Conjunctivitis. *Clinical Evidence* 4: 350–355.

Khaw PT, Elkington AR (1999). *ABC of Eyes*. London: BMJ.

Li Wan Po A (1990). *Non-Prescription Drugs* (2nd edn). Oxford: Blackwell Scientific Publications.

Martini FH (2001). *Fundamentals of Anatomy and Physiology* (5th edn). Upper Saddle River: Prentice Hall.

Porth CM (1994). *Pathophysiology: Concepts of Altered Health States* (4th edn). Philadelphia: JB Lippincott.

Serra AM, Bailey CM, Jackson P (1986). *Ear, Nose and Throat Nursing*. Oxford: Blackwell Scientific Publications.

Sullivan JH, Crawford JB, Whitcher JP (1999). In: Vaughn D, Ashbury T, Riordan-Eva P (eds). *General Opthalmology* (15th edn). Stamford: Appleton and Lange.

Tullo AB, Donnelly D (1995). Conjunctiva. In: Perry JP, Tullo AB (eds). *Care of the Opthalmic Patient – A Guide for Nurses and Health Professionals* (2nd edn). London: Chapman and Hall.

Chapter 11

Products and Preparations for Minor Ailments of the Circulatory System

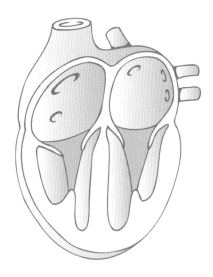

This chapter provides an overview of the circulatory system including the respiratory and venous pump systems. Superficial phlebitis, the role of NSAIDs and compression therapy in the treatment management of this condition is then described.

The Circulatory System

Blood flows through the body in a closed network called the circulatory system. From the left ventricle, blood passes into the aorta and then into other arteries. Arteries carry the blood away from the heart. Each artery branches approximately 15–20 times, becoming smaller and smaller. These small arteries are called arterioles, which lead into a network of minute capillaries. Oxygen and nutrients diffuse through the thin walls of these vessels into the tissues of the body. The capillaries eventually form venules, which lead onto veins. Veins take the blood back to the right atrium. The right ventricle then pumps this blood to the lungs where it becomes oxygenated, and then it returns to the left side of the heart. The blood therefore has two journeys: around the body in the systemic circulation, and to the lungs and back in the pulmonary circulation. At any one time, three quarters of the blood is in veins, one-fifth in arteries, and one-twentieth in capillaries.

The Structure of Blood Vessels

Arteries and veins are composed of three layers:

- *Tunica adventia* – This layer is the outermost layer of the vessel and forms a connective tissue sheath. This sheath helps to stabilise and anchor the vessel by the blending of connective tissue fibres into adjacent tissue. In veins, the tunica adventia is generally thicker than the tunica media.

- *Tunica media* – This layer consists of involuntary muscle, which is stimulated by sympathetic nerve fibres, and elastic fibres. It is responsible for the change in lumen size of the vessel, and is very thick in arteries. In vasodilation, the muscle is relaxed and the vessel open. In vasoconstriction, the muscle contracts, and the vessel narrows. Collagen fibres within the tunica media bind it to the tunica adventia and tunica intima.

- *Tunica intima* – This layer is comprised of a smooth lining of endothelial cells, which also forms the valves, and a basement membrane.

Blood vessels are designed in such a way as to function effectively in their specific roles (Figure 11.1). Capillaries are comprised of a single layer of cells, and so allow the easy passage of oxygen and nutrients into the surrounding tissue. Arteries have very thick muscular walls, enabling them to cope with the high-pressure surges of blood from the heart. Veins have loose, slack walls as the blood in them is under very little pressure.

Figure 11.1 – Structure of blood vessels

Artery

Vein

Tunica adventitia

Lumen

Lumen

Tunica media

Tunica intima

Tunica intima

Capillary

Single layer of endothelial cells

Nucleus of endothelial cell

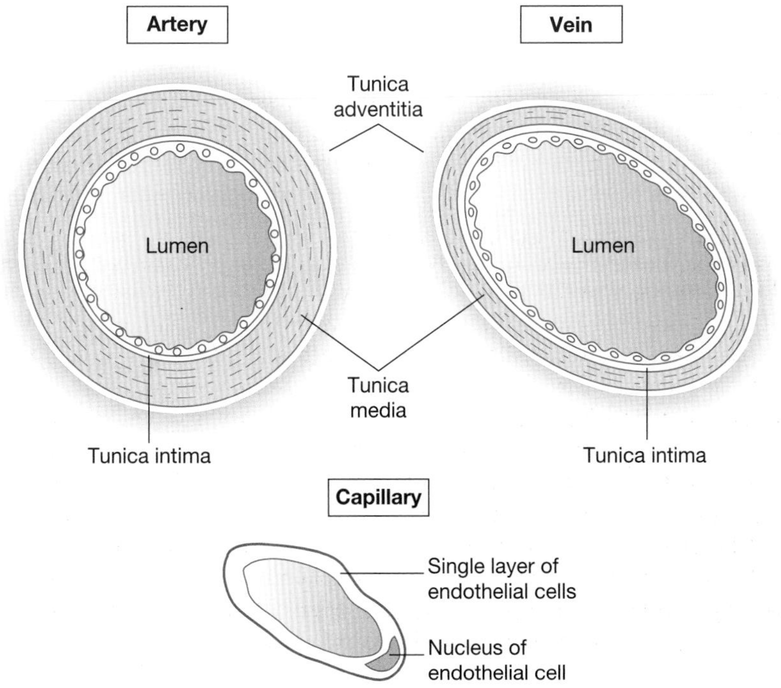

Venous return

The pressure in the venous system determines the volume of blood returned to the heart. This is directly related to cardiac output and peripheral blood flow. To maintain cardiac output, the venous blood has to travel through a complex vascular network. However, the blood pressure at the beginning of the venous system is approximately ten times less than at the start of the arterial system.

Three input mechanisms are involved in the return of the venous blood to the heart:

- The respiratory pump
- The venous pump
- Venous valves

The respiratory pump

The thoracic cavity expands as a person inhales and the pressure within the pleural cavities is reduced. This drop in pressure causes air to be pulled into the lungs. At the same time, blood is also pulled from the smaller veins of the abdominal cavity and lower body into the inferior vena cava and right atrium. During exhalation, the thoracic cavity is decreased in size. Thus the internal pressure is caused to rise. Air is forced out of the lungs, and venous blood pushed into the right atrium.

The venous pump

The venous system of the leg (Figure 11.2), comprises:

- The femoral, popliteal, and tibial deep veins encased and supported by the tough, deep fascia muscle sheath.
- The long and short saphenous superficia veins lying outside the fascia.
- The short perforator connecting veins perforate the fascia.

The pressure of the blood in the leg veins results from the weight of the blood itself and is highest at the lowest point. When an individual is standing still, the pressure of the blood in the deep veins of the foot is approximately 90 mmHg. This pressure is much lower in the superficial veins and capillaries.

During normal standing and walking, the venous pump assists venous return. As the calf muscles contract, they become shorter and thicker and compress nearby blood vessels propelling blood towards the heart. During muscle relaxation, the vessel once again fills with blood and the cycle is repeated during the next contraction. When a person is standing still for a long period of time, the venous pump does not operate and blood pools in the legs.

Venous valves

The valves, present in leg veins, play a crucial role in the efficiency of the venous pump. Valves are formed from the endothelial lining of the tunica intima and are semi-lunar folds that point in the direction of blood flow. The valves in the leg veins have a similar action to the valves in the heart. They allow blood to flow in one direction only, and prevent it from flowing back towards the capillaries. Therefore, any movement that distorts or compresses a vein will push blood

Figure 11.2 – Venous system of the leg

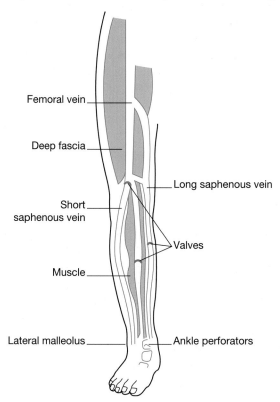

Femoral vein

Deep fascia

Long saphenous vein

Short saphenous vein

Valves

Muscle

Lateral malleolus

Ankle perforators

towards the heart. Without valves, the effects of gravity when standing upright would cause pooling of blood in the leg veins and fail to overcome the pull of gravity to ascend to the heart.

The blood is compartmentalised by valves. Therefore, the weight of the blood is divided between each of the compartments in the vein. Movement in the surrounding skeletal muscle squeezes the blood towards the heart. When standing, very fast cycles of contraction and relaxation occur within the leg muscles, the contractions pushing the blood towards the heart. When lying down, the heart and major vessels are at the same level. Therefore, venous valves have much less impact on venous return.

The valves in the perforator connecting veins have the most important role. If these valves fail to work effectively, the high pressure in the deep veins, is transmitted to the much weaker, unsupported superficial veins. These veins become distended and tortuous (varicose veins). Capillary pressure becomes increased, and fluid is forced out into the extravascular space. This can then progress onto chronic venous insufficiency characterised by oedema, pigmentation, eczema, and ulceration of the leg.

Superficial phlebitis

Inflammation of the vein walls, or phlebitis, usually occurs following an injury to the vein which produces and inflammatory response in the vessel wall. It is apt to arise in circumstances in which there is stasis in the leg veins and is a common complication of varicose veins. Venous thrombosis, i.e. clot formation in a vein often occurs secondary to phlebitis. Superficial phlebitis presents as a marked redness, tenderness, and swelling along the course of the vein. Other symptoms may include fever, lymphangitis, and systemic upset (MCA, 2001). Heat, NSAIDs and compression stockings are used to treat uncomplicated, superficial thrombophlebitis.

Preparations for the treatment of superficial phlebitis:

- Ibuprofen granules 600 mg/sachet and syrup 100 mg/5 ml (Brufen®)
- Ibuprofen modified release tablets and capsules 800 mg (Brufen Retard®)
- Ibuprofen tablets 200 mg, 400 mg, 600 mg, 800 mg, and suspension 100 mg/1 ml (Brufen®)

For mode of action, contraindications, adverse effects, and nursing points *see* Chapter 3.

Compression Therapy

Compression therapy applies graduated compression from the toe base to the knee. The application of pressure is highest at the ankle. This is reduced by at least 50% at the knee (Moffatt, 1992). This constant graded pressure encourages the complete emptying of veins, decreasing venous pooling, and venous stasis. Compression hosiery is one method of achieving graduated compression.

Compression hosiery

Thigh length, below knee stockings, socks, and tights are all styles of compression hosiery available. Items conform to the British Standards Institution (BSI) and come in made-to-measure and standard sizes. Manufacturers also offer different combinations of colour and open or closed heels or toes. Stockings are classified according to the maximum pressure at the ankle and the pressure gradients at calf and thigh (Figure 11.3). Standard methods are in place for batch testing of these garments, and an important attribute is durability. Following 30 washes, in accordance with the manufacturers instructions, the stockings have to maintain 85% of their original pressure.

Classes

There are three different classes of compression hosiery. Each class differs with regard to the level of pressure exerted. The classes, as described by the National Health Service Drug Tariff (2001), are as follows:

- *Class I* – This class provides light (mild) support and produces compression of 14–17 mmHg at the ankle.

  Indications: These stockings are for superficial or early varices and those occurring during pregnancy.

Figure 11.3 – Compression gradients in graduated compression hosiery (Modified from Kemp, 1996)

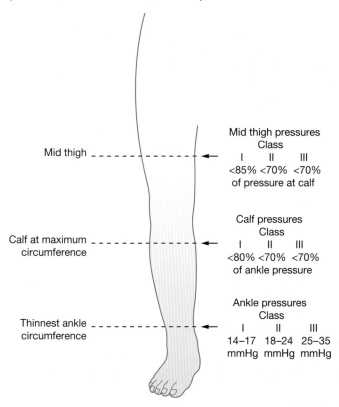

Mid thigh

Mid thigh pressures
Class

I	II	III
<85%	<70%	<70%

of pressure at calf

Calf at maximum
circumference

Calf pressures
Class

I	II	III
<80%	<70%	<70%

of ankle pressure

Thinnest ankle
circumference

Ankle pressures
Class

I	II	III
14–17 mmHg	18–24 mmHg	25–35 mmHg

- *Class II* – These stockings provide medium (moderate) support. Compression at the ankle is 18–24 mmHg.

  Indications: They are generally used for varices of medium severity, ulcer treatment and prevention of recurrence, mild oedema, varicosis during pregnancy, and for soft tissue support.

- *Class III* – These stockings provide strong support. Compression at the ankle is 25–35 mmHg.

  Indications: This class is used for gross varices, post-thrombotic venous insufficiency, gross oedema, ulcer treatment and prevention of recurrence, and soft tissue support.

Types

The different types of compression stockings are described by Kemp (1996). These include:

- Circular knit
- Flat-bed knit stockings

- Net stockings
- One-way stretch stockings (Class III only)

Each different type of stocking is made of a different material. Circular knit stockings are made of nylon and cotton yarn. These stockings are available as a made-to-measure item and in standard sizes. However, their lack of stretch makes them difficult to apply. Flat-bed stockings are made of cotton, nylon, and nylon-plated varieties and offer greater flexibility but, are only available on prescription as a made-to-measure item. Net stockings, are seamed and made of a net fabric. Although often the least cosmetically acceptable, they are useful if a patients leg is an unusual shape. However, this type of stocking is only available as a made-to-measure item. One-way stretch stockings are also a made-to-measure item. These stockings are without a seam (apart from at the toe and the heel) and are made of a heavy circular machine knit.

The selection of compression hosiery

The style of stocking should be determined in the initial assessment. Kemp (1996) has identified a number of factors that influence the type and style of stocking selected.

These include:

- The patient's age
- The dexterity of the patient
- Whether or not the patient is disabled
- The condition of the patient's skin
- The appearance of the stocking
- The type of hosiery the patient normally wears and the mode of suspension

An important point that must be considered is the dexterity of the patient. Thigh length compression hosiery can be difficult to apply correctly and below knee hosiery might be a better choice.

Measuring for elastic hosiery

Measurements of the patient's leg should take place early in the morning or, following a period of leg elevation. This will ensure that the effects of oedema are kept to a minimum.

For standard size knee stockings, the following measurements must be taken:

- The ankle circumference of the patient at the thinnest point
- The calf circumference at the widest point
- The below knee length

If the patient requires thigh length standard stockings, the measurements are the same as for below knee stockings, but also including the mid-thigh circumference and leg length.

Made-to-measure hosiery

If standard hosiery does not fit the patient, they will need made-to-measure garments. Figure 11.4 highlights the points on the leg where measurements should be taken.

Figure 11.4 – Points on the leg where measurements should be taken for made-to-measure garments (Modified from Kemp, 1996)

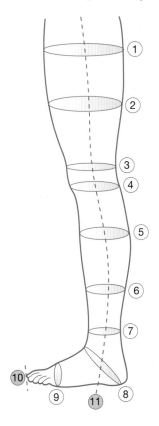

Circumference
1. Top of thigh
2. Mid point between 1 and 3
3. Knee at widest point
4. Base of knee, i.e. point where below knee stocking ends
5. Widest calf circumference
6. Midpoint between 5 and 7
7. Ankle at narrowest point if it is not possible to identify this point measure 2–4 cm above ankle bone
8. Widest point for stocking to pass
9. Toe base-note any abnormalities

Length
10 to 8 and 9 to 6-draw around the clients foot whilst they are standing on paper. Mark the widest point at toe base (position 9)
11. Point that measurement must be made between the height of each circumference and the floor

Prescribing elastic hosiery

Before the prescription for elastic hosiery can be dispensed, the following details must be provided by the prescriber:

- The quantity – single or pair
- The article, i.e. style and type including any accessories
- Compression Class I, II, or III
- Patient measurements if stockings are to be made-to-measure

Fitting elastic hosiery

Most patients will need to be shown how to apply compression hosiery. The following points need to be considered:

- When applying stockings, turn the stocking inside out to the heel. Thumbs should then be inserted into the sides of the stocking and the stocking applied. The heel must be in the correct position. Ease the stocking up the ankle and leg. Spread the stocking evenly ensuring there are no tight bands. The stocking must be reapplied if it is pulled up too high.

- A silky socklet which is supplied by the manufacturer will ease the application of open-toed stockings.
- Stockings must be taken off at night and reapplied first thing in the morning. This will ensure that oedema has not collected.
- To avoid feelings of claustrophobia, patients may, at first, only be able to tolerate compression stockings for short periods of time.
- It may be necessary to re-measure the patient's leg after a few weeks if the hosiery has been effective in reducing oedema.
- Although aids may be helpful when applying elastic hosiery, it may be necessary, depending upon patient dexterity, to seek the help of a relative or friend.
- If a patient is unable to apply Class III stockings, it might be more appropriate to wear two pairs of Class I, stocking as pressure is cumulative (Fentem, 1986).

Washing elastic hosiery

Clear washing instructions are provided with compression hosiery. Items should be handwashed at 40°C. Frequent daily washing improves performance by restoring shape and removing skin oils. If cared for correctly, stockings should provide adequate pressure for 3 or 4 months before needing to be replaced.

Contraindications (Elastic hosiery)

Patients suffering from severe arteriosclerosis or any other ischaemic vascular disease should not wear compression hosiery. Stockings should also be avoided if any local conditions affecting the leg, e.g. skin lesions, gangrenous conditions, or recent vein ligation, are present. In these situations they may compromise the circulation.

Allergies due to the stocking fibres are rare. However, if a patient has a very sensitive skin, a patch test should be performed. A sample of the stocking can be obtained from the manufacturer.

Haemorrhoids

Haemorrhoids or piles, are varices in the veins of the ano-rectal canal. These enlarged, dilated, and displaced vascular cushions arise as a result of elevated venous pressure. Unable to resist the pressure, the walls of the veins stretch and dilate. Common causes include straining at the stool when constipated, and pregnancy (both of which increase abdominopelvic cavity pressure).

Travis *et al.* (1998) classifies haemorrhoids using descriptive terms rather than the traditional classification. These terms include: bleeding, temporarily or permanently prolapsed, and thrombosed.

Bleeding

This commonly appears as bright red blood around the toilet pan after defaecation. Blood may also smear the outside of the stool. Individuals complaining of bleeding require medical assessment as rectal carcinoma and other causes of rectal bleeding need to be excluded.

Prolapse
The patient recognises prolapse and the haemorrhoids can be visualised by the attending nurse or physician. They typically appear as tender, painful, blue-coloured, localised swellings in the peri-anal region. The prolapse has to be distinguished from a polyp, rectal prolapse, anal tumour or skin tag.

Thrombosis
This is of rapid onset and causes severe peri-anal pain. Medical attention is required.

(Travis *et al.*, 1998)

Patients with haemorrhoids should be given advice to prevent straining and constipation. This should include information about the importance of a high fibre diet. Non-operative measures for the management of haemorrhoids include the prescription of suppositories and ointments, which have little more than a placebo effect (Hancock, 1999). Corticosteroids may be combined with local anaesthetics, and soothing preparations containing mild astringents, in preparation for the treatment of haemorrhoids. Peri-anal thrush must be excluded before using these products.

Preparations for the treatment of haemorrhoids:

- Anugesic-HC® cream and suppositories
- Anusol-HC® ointment and suppositories
- Betnovate® rectal ointment
- Cinchocaine and Hydrocortisone ointment and suppositories (Proctosedyl®)
- Cinchocaine and Prednisolone ointment and suppositories (Scheriproct®)
- Hydrocortisone and Pramocaine rectal foam (Proctofoam HC®)
- Ultraproct® ointment and suppositories
- Xyloproct® ointment

The reader should consult Chapter 6 for the mode of action, contraindications, adverse effects, and nursing points related to topical corticosteroids.

Mode of action
Local anaesthetics such as lidocaine, cinchocaine, and pramocaine are used to prevent pain and discomfort associated with haemorrhoids, though good evidence is lacking. They cause a reversible block of conduction along nerve fibres to produce both a loss of sensation and a loss of muscle activity. Small, non-myelinated pain fibres are most sensitive to these drugs, and are the first to be depressed. Subsequent loss of function of other types of nerves then occurs. The drug is administered at the desired site of action and penetrates the inside of the nerve axon, binding to receptors in the sodium channels. This results in these channels becoming blocked (Figure 11.5). Ultimately, depolarisation of the cell membrane is prevented, action potentials are not generated, and the nerve

Figure 11.5 – Local anaesthetic drug blocking a sodium channel

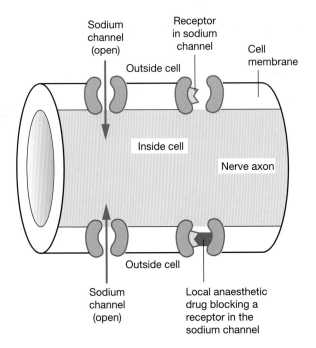

becomes 'blocked'. The inhibition of nerve conduction persists until the drug diffuses and enters the circulation for subsequent metabolism and excretion.

Contraindications

Caution should be taken if patients have cardiovascular or central nervous system problems. Excessive use of local anaesthetics may lead to systemic problems.

Adverse effects

Skin rash, due to local allergy, may occur with chronic use. Excessive application may result in increased absorption through the rectal mucosa, and systemic adverse effects. These may include convulsions, paraesthesia, nervousness, tremors, hypotension, and bradycardia. These products should be used for short periods only, and avoided in infants and children.

Nursing Points

Most haemorrhoidal preparations should not be used for longer than 7 days. They are usually applied twice daily and/or after bowel movements. The patient should be referred to a physician where there are complaints of anal/rectal bleeding and where the diagnosis is unclear.

References

Drug Tarriff (2001). National Health Service England and Wales. London: The Stationery Office.

Fentem PH (1986). Elastic hosiery. *Pharmacy Update* 5: 200–205.

Hancock BD (1999). Haemorrhoids. In: Jones DJ (ed). *ABC of Colorectal Diseases* (2nd edn). London: BMJ.

Kemp D (1996). Compression hosiery. *Professional Nurse* 11(10) 697–700.

MCA (2001). *Extended Prescribing of Prescription Only Medicines By Independent Nurse Prescribers*. London: MCA.

Moffatt CJ (1992). Compression bandaging: the state of the art. *J Wound Care* 1(1) 45–50.

Travis SPL, Taylor RH, Misiewicz JJ (1998). *Gastroenterology*. (2nd edn). Oxford: Blackwell Science.

INDEX

Note: Drugs are listed by their generic name but not their trade name (except for rare exceptions where their generic equivalent is not mentioned).
Abbreviations: COC, combined oral contraceptive; POP, progesterone-only pill.